Alcohol Use

Radcliffe Medical Press

D1339781

£19.95

Radcliffe Medical Press Ltd
18 Marcham Road, Abingdon, Oxon OX14 1AA

British Library Cataloguing in Publication Data

A catalogue record for this book is available from the British Library.

ISBN 1 85775 121 3

Typeset by The Midlands Book Typesetting Company, Leicestershire
Printed and bound by TJ International Ltd, Padstow, Cornwall

Contents

List of contributors

Salme Ahlström, Research Professor, Alcohol and Drug Research, National Research and Development Centre for Welfare and Health, Helsinki, Finland

Karin L Anseline, Lecturer and Private Consultant, Hawks Nest, New South Wales, Australia

Anne E Bartu, Principal Research Officer, Next Step Specialist Drug and Alcohol Services and Senior Lecturer, Curtin University of Technology, Perth, Australia

Terry C Blum, Tedd Munchak Professor of Management and Dean of the Du Pree College of Management, Georgia Institute of Technology, Atlanta, Georgia, USA

Douglas Cameron, Senior Lecturer (Clinical) in Substance Misuse, University of Leicester; Honorary Consultant Psychiatrist, Leicestershire NHS Drug and Alcohol Service, Leicester, UK

Paul Clenaghan, Project Coordinator – Mental Health, Manley Hospital, Manley, New South Wales, Australia

David B Cooper, Freelance Author, Editor and Consultant, Chulmleigh, Devon, UK

J Aaron Johnson, Project Coordinator, Institute for Behavioral Research, University of Georgia, USA

Ian MacEwan, Manager – Treatment Development, Alcohol Advisory Council of New Zealand, Wellington, New Zealand

Eileen McKee, Executive Director, COPA, Toronto, Ontario, Canada

Olga Maranjian Church, Professor and Project Director, Addiction Training Center of New England: Nursing, University of Connecticut, USA

Marjana Martinic, Director of Science Policy, International Center for Alcohol Policies, Washington, DC, USA

Pip Mason, Freelance Trainer, Kings Norton, Birmingham, UK

Theresa B Moyers, Research Professor, University of New Mexico, Albuquerque, USA

Alex Paton, Consultant Physician, Chadlington, Oxon, UK

Paul M Roman, Research Professor of Sociology and Director, Center for Research on Behavioral Health and Human Service Delivery, Institute for Behavioral Research, University of Georgia, USA

Susan A Storti, Director, Addiction Technology Transfer Center of New England, Brown University, Providence, USA

Richard Velleman, Professor of Mental Health Research and Director, Research and Development Unit, University of Bath, UK

Hazel E Watson, Senior Lecturer, Department of Nursing, Glasgow Caledonian University City Campus, UK

USA foreword

In the United States, alcohol dependence is the most common chronic illness between the ages of 18 and 44, and its impact on the US economy has been estimated at $98.6 billion. In addition, between 25–40% of all general hospital patients are there because of complications related to alcohol use. I venture to say that the US is not alone among nations with this pervasive problem. Yet despite a growing global awareness that alcohol may be the most commonly used drug, it is also the least understood.

The United Nation's declaration of the years 1991–2000 as the 'decade against drugs' inspired global involvement in the development of behavioural, epidemiological, economical and biomedical initiatives in research and education. The need to disseminate the findings continues and the challenge to provide clear and relevant resources has been successfully met by the Editor of this book.

David B Cooper's commitment to inform health professionals on a wide spectrum of issues related to behavioural health and addictions in general, and alcohol use in particular, is well known in the field. As editor of the widely acclaimed *Journal of Substance Use*, he provided a welcome forum for a broad spectrum of educators, researchers and practitioners. Together with the authors and contributors to this book, Cooper offers the novice an in-depth and practical orientation to the field of substance use. As a practical guide about the problems inherent in alcohol use and the possibilities for intervention, the book also serves to update practitioners in their search for timely and effective approaches in caring for this client group.

The impact of alcohol use at various points along the life span as well as a variety of treatment and therapeutic options are addressed in this book. In addition, multiple learning devices such as interactive exercises, self-assessment tools and case studies enhance the engagement of the reader. The authors, providing the reader with a variety of national perspectives, address such diverse and important areas as transcultural, workplace and community issues.

It has been said that the most lasting ways to affect public opinion, knowledge, attitudes and beliefs is through a heightened awareness. Transforming that awareness into appropriate clinical and social approaches to alcohol use remains a complicated task. Healthcare professionals everywhere should feel encouraged by this book and the promise it offers for informed and effective care.

Olga Maranjian Church
Professor and Project Director
Addiction Training Center
University of Connecticut
April 2000

UK foreword

The invitation to write a foreword to a book is always a compliment. To be invited to write a foreword to a book on alcohol use is almost like an invitation to join the editor at the bar. I was flattered to receive the invitation and I wish David and all his contributors the 'very best of health' as I symbolically raise my glass to their good fortunes and that of this important book.

The invitation to write the foreword to a book about alcohol use requires some reflection on one's own use of the Devil's drink, or *usquebaugh*, as my Celtic forebears would rather have called it – for what else might something like whisky be, but the *water of life*. I am somewhat alarmed to recall that I was 30 before I ever 'touched a drop' of anything alcoholic. Moreover, the first time I can recall being even the slightest bit 'merry' was at my daughter's 18th birthday party, by which time I was nearer to 40. Why the long wait, I ask myself. Perhaps I was more fearful of my Celtic roots, and all that wild, reckless enjoyment of life – which included just a few pints and drams – than I was actually fearful of the drink itself. Certainly my grandfather and my father both 'enjoyed' a drink, but were never its victims. Perhaps I was just slow to enjoy the comforts of 'enjoyment'. Most people who develop a problem with alcohol, in either overfondness or aversion, have good historical reasons for it. I certainly had no such reasons. My teetotalism was probably rooted in pomposity, in a certain kind of high-mindedness, in – dare I say – a Calvinistic outlook on life. I am glad now that I managed to break with all those self-imposed rules about drink and drinkers. In so doing I allowed myself the opportunity to share one last drink with my dying father, in a wee pub on the Kirkcaldy esplanade, after he had steeled himself to endure one more of those pointless, impersonal examinations of his cancerous chest. I recall that his eyes sparkled for the first time in at least a year as he finished his second pint and said 'time for home, son!' My memory may be playing tricks with me, but I do recall him trying to compensate for the uncertainty of his gait, with a little hop and skip, as I had seen him do many times before as he headed home from the Ex-serviceman's Club. It cheered my heart to see him just a little 'under the weather'. At least he was living out his final days in the same way as he had tried to live his major years: celebrating life and companionship, knowing that, like the glass, what once was full would soon be emptied. As I cleared the dregs of my own glass, I silently thanked myself for allowing my father to model one of the useful 'uses' of alcohol before it was too late: oiling the wheels of social intercourse, a means to an end rather than an end in itself.

My thoughts turn first to my father and my own slow introduction to the pleasures of alcohol, for clearly David B Cooper's book is about alcohol *use*. It is not a negative treatise on alcohol. It is not even a book about alcohol *ab*use. It is certainly not an anti-alcohol book. It is an intelligent and balanced reflection on an important dimension of our personal and social lives: one that can thankfully be assessed, for most of us, as a useful means to a very useful social end. For others, alcohol can signal the rise and fall of all kinds of problems: personal, social and cultural. Indeed, the signalling function of alcohol use can hardly be overstated. How we use alcohol – or indeed, choose not to use it – can tell us so much about who we are, where we stand in our personal and social development, even our location – as individuals – within the whirl of our social and cultural milieu. It would not be praising this book too highly to suggest that the appreciation of alcohol use conveyed by the authors helps to locate us *spiritually* in the post-modern world; where so much is known but so little is understood. Given that it can signal so many of these dimensions of our personal and social world, we all should treat the *usquebaugh* with, at least, some reverence. Alcohol – like many other objects of our construction – is of good character. It is only our *use* of this child of our creation that can become problematic.

Before we reflect on the perils and pitfalls of alcohol use we should not forget how important alcohol use has been, not only for us in the simple social sense, but as an aid to creative powers of many writers, poets and artists. Careful use of alcohol has helped many people to manage the demons within their souls and, in some cases, has at the same time freed them to experience some of their full humanness that those demons originally denied them. Some of those people would argue that alcohol was a *necessary* adjunct to artistic creation. Whether alcohol was *sufficient* – in itself – to produce great art is less convincing. The lyrical beauty of a Dylan Thomas poem, or the expressionistic energy of a Jackson Pollock canvas, may have been facilitated by a few drinks, but could never be attributed to the work of the *usquebaugh* itself. Making such fine distinctions is central to the mission of this book. Few of us will aspire to create great works of art. For us lesser mortals alcohol use will serve a lower order function: encouraging us to believe that after a few drinks we *can* be more sociable, feel less insecure, sense an elevation of our human spirits. Herein lies the key to alcohol use: that by careful use, we may appreciate more of our world and ourselves, but in overuse we might lose our grasp of both those dimensions of our human experience. How people have, and continue to, judge the boundary between careful and overuse of this sparkling child of our creation is a lesson worth learning. Like all lessons, we can learn much from the painfulness of our own experience but also much from the pain and success of others.

David B Cooper's book represents a valuable vehicle for learning the trick of alcohol use: how knowledge about alcohol might empower us and how that knowledge might take away some of the fear that might make us vulnerable to the *usquebaugh*. David and his colleagues illustrate just how rich is the seam of alcohol knowledge, and have done the field of alcohol abuse a great service in the production of this richly varied account on the oldest of our substance abuse scenarios. They have also modelled a positive outlook, by concerned professionals, to the wider world of alcohol use. The world of alcohol use – and abuse – sorely needs some positive, authoritative voices. I am confident that I shall be empowered by returning to consider carefully the many lessons contained within this text. I wish them every success in their endeavour to enrichen everyone's knowledge and experience of relating to the *usquebaugh*. That is an endeavour well worth toasting. *Slainthé.*

Phil Barker
Professor of Psychiatric Nursing Practice
University of Newcastle
April 2000

Preface

Humanity has a long-standing love–hate relationship with the beverage alcohol. Alcohol is consumed in most countries. Its use in many societies is both widespread and deeply rooted in tradition. In others its consumption has been more restricted, but appears to be increasing due to social changes and commercial pressures.[1] Most of those who drink alcohol generally do so in moderation and without any adverse consequences. Indeed, most drinkers' lives are enhanced by alcohol consumption and some even derive a degree of health benefit from it. The latter is mainly in the form of reduced rates of cardiovascular disease amongst older people who are light drinkers. Sadly, some people do, on occasion, drink in ways which are risky, inappropriate and harmful. Some do so only rarely, while others do so routinely and chronically. Some people become alcohol dependent ('alcoholic'), while far more experience a constellation of adverse effects such as illness, accident, public disorder, social, employment or other difficulties. Heavy drinking is not only risky, it can and does sometimes kill. Even so, alcohol-related problems are not necessarily intractable, either at the individual level or social level. There are many examples of ways in which both individuals with such problems can be helped through the difficult periods of their lives and of how communities may reduce the level of trouble associated with heavy or inappropriate drinking.[2,3]

The consumption of alcohol, like other commonplace social activities, has attracted comment for centuries. Even so, during the past three decades there has been an explosion in the amount of scientific inquiry and discussion into every conceivable aspect of what has been called 'our favourite drug'.[4]

The amount of information about alcohol consumption and its ramifications is now so vast that no single person can possibly read, let alone absorb, it all. Many of those who are professionally involved with alcohol issues find it hard to keep up with even developments and evidence related to their specialist areas of concern. Few of those in the health and social services, for example, have either the resources, time or inclination to wade through esoteric specialist journals. Accordingly, there is a pressing need for texts such as *Alcohol Use*. This provides the reader with a coherent, concise and balanced overview of some of the main topics that are likely to interest many of those with an interest in alcohol issues.

The production of this book is timely. A lot of information, which has accumulated over the past decade, has cast new light on a number of key issues. Some of these are epidemiological. Others relate to clinical subjects. These include evidence about the protective effects of low alcohol consumption, the consumption of alcohol by elderly people, transcultural issues and the merits of alternative and sometimes relatively inexpensive ways of providing help and support for those who experience alcohol-related problems.

This book presents a wide-ranging array of information in an accessible and digestible form. The international team of contributors (from Australia, Canada, Finland, New Zealand, the UK and the USA) is well chosen, being experienced and authoritative about their selected topics. The first part of the book, Chapters 2–11, is broadly concerned with general/epidemiological issues and sets the scene for the second part which is focused on responses to alcohol-related problems. The initial chapters discuss alcohol use in perspective, alcohol and the body, alcohol and the young adult, man and woman, the family, the older person, mental health and mental illness, transcultural issues and the workplace. These contributions are informative and clear. They offer the reader a user-friendly overview based upon a fair review of available evidence. These reviews are enlivened by balanced and perceptive comment. The latter is evidence-driven, rather than ideology-driven. This is important and is to be commended in a field in which rhetoric and ideology sometimes obscure both the evidence and its implications.

The second part of the book deals with issues such as prevention, identification, education and health promotion. Thereafter, the text concentrates on clinical and other practical concerns. These include change and motivation, assessment, alcohol detoxification, other therapeutic interventions, creating common ground and the need for professional communication. The text concludes with a thought-provoking commentary by the Editor entitled 'Conclusion: entering the room'. This serves as a useful reminder that scientific evidence in this complex field should constantly be subject to review and reappraisal.

The material presented provides an excellent and digestible guide through important subject areas, which would otherwise take a long time to begin to penetrate in any sensible way. The contributors perform a valuable service here for those who might wish to obtain an informed and intelligent overview of important issues related to prevention, clinical approaches and other constructive and effective ways of responding to alcohol problems. They also present a useful introduction to the social/psychological setting in which such problems develop and need to be handled.

David B Cooper is to be congratulated on assembling an original and valuable addition to the alcohol literature. He has already made a major contribution in this respect, both through his own writings[5] and through his role as editor-in-chief of the *Journal of Substance Use.*

Alcohol Use is intended to be of particular value as an introductory text for those who are new to the field. In fact, it provides a very useful collection of reviews that would also be of great value to many of those who have worked in the field a long time. All such people periodically need to update their basic knowledge. This book should be on the shelf of anyone with a professional or personal serious interest in this fascinating, important and enduring aspect of the human condition.

Martin Plant
Director
Alcohol and Health Research Centre
City Hospital
Edinburgh
April 2000

Acknowledgements

I am grateful to all the authors, Dr Martin Plant, Professor Phil Barker, Professor Olga Maranjian Church and those who have commented on or contributed to the book in a large or small way throughout its formative years, completion and publication. Each author is to be commended for their hard work, dedication and patience throughout this period. Any success the book may have will be due to their knowledge, experience and commitment and the fact that each one of the authors cares enough to want to work with, and for, the individual who experiences problems with alcohol use. Any errors, omissions or deficiencies within these pages are the sole responsibility of the editor.

I am also grateful to the people who have influenced my time in the substance use field. Whilst I can name only a few, I would like to thank them all. I am particularly grateful to Martin and Moira Plant, who have always been encouraging, genuine and supportive. Martin, David Peck and Jonathan Chick were all extremely helpful and encouraging when my first rather poor attempts at research, and its written presentation, arrived unsolicited on their desks in 1984–85! Doug Cameron, Olga Maranjian Church, Richard Pates and Paul Stoneman have all contributed to my knowledge, thinking, practice and learning. Phil Barker, Philip Burnard, Keith Yoxhall and many more influenced, directly or indirectly, my work and clinical practice. I am also very much indebted to Louise Sallis, formerly of Radcliffe Medical Press, who encouraged, cared and prodded in a helpful way throughout the book's journey to publication: Gillian Nineham, whose words 'we'll get there in the end' have now come true – at last – and to Heidi Allen and Jamie Etherington who continued and completed the challenge! Thank you to Jo, who has been involved with the project throughout and is always supportive and encouraging, whatever the ideas! My sincere thanks and appreciation to all of you, named and unnamed.

This book is dedicated to the memory
of Albert Edwin Harvey, a gentle man,
to Joyce and Charlie Cooper, who are
always there to support, and to my children
Phil, Marc and Caroline. All, in their very
special ways, have influenced my life for
the better. It is also dedicated, with my
love, to Jo, a special person who has
unquestioning faith, trust, support and
love, all the time. Her encouragement
makes the ideas and notions progress
to fruition, and for that I thank
her unreservedly.

CHAPTER 1

Introduction:
opening the door

David B Cooper

Pre-reading preparation

When preparing to read this book you may wish to undertake the following exercise.

Write a brief description of your thoughts and feelings in relation to alcohol use and alcohol-related problems.

When you have read the book, you may wish to repeat the exercise, taking note of the following:

• Have your thoughts and feelings changed?
• If yes, in what way?
• What information do you feel most influenced this change?
• Are there any areas that you feel you need to investigate further?
• If yes, what are they? What resources could you use?

If you would like to comment on the book, please write to the editor:

Mr David B Cooper,
Parkholme,
Ashreigney,
Chulmleigh,
Devon,
EX18 7LY,
UK.

Your opinions are important and welcome.

In 1980, this author, then a newly qualified staff nurse working on a 25-bed acute admission ward, was approached to 'run the alcoholic group'. The group had been about to meet for the first time when the nurse in charge left the authority for career advancement. Approximately 10 people were due to attend the first session, and there were no willing takers to run the group. Naively (or arrogantly), this author agreed. It was immediately apparent that the two-hour lecture listened to during nurse training was useless. The decision was easy – if this author's contribution was to be in any way meaningful and therapeutic then more training, education and knowledge were needed. The learning curve was sharp! Interestingly, but not surprisingly, the move to educate this novice came from the individuals who were supposed to be benefiting from his 'therapeutic interventions'. That is, those individuals who attended that group provided this author with an understanding of the nature of *their* problems.

Obtaining in-depth and knowledgeable text on treatment was not difficult. However, one had to trawl a broad spectrum of work to find out the basics – the background details that one needs on which to build professional practice. It was apparent that what was needed was a basic text, in one book, that would introduce this first, but vital, step into the field of alcohol use.

The opportunity to bring about such a publication, where leaders from the alcohol field have agreed to share their specialist knowledge, has been an ambition for many years. Now, it is no longer a dream. It is hoped that this publication will assist the reader to take the first step towards an understanding of alcohol use and alcohol-related problems.

The book is intended for those new to the field of substance use. It is written on the assumption that in order to meet the needs of those experiencing alcohol-related problems, health, social, legal and spiritual care professionals need a basic introduction, education and training in the practice and management of alcohol use prevention, identification, brief intervention and support services.

This is not an anti-alcohol book. It is very much a practical, basic guide about the problems alcohol use can cause some individuals, the types of intervention required, and addressing problems the individual encounters. The term 'use', rather than 'misuse' or 'abuse', will be used in recognition that many individuals with problems arising from the use of alcohol, with whom the target readership have contact, will consider their use 'normal'. That is, not associated with the physical, legal, social or psychological problems they are presenting with.

The book offers a first-step introduction, relevant to the needs of the professional, in a clear, concise and understandable format. Each chapter has made full use of boxes, graphs, tables, interactive exercises, self-assessment tools and case studies, where appropriate, to examine and demonstrate the effect alcohol use can have on the individual, the family and society as a whole. The book also looks at various treatments and therapeutic interventions available and concludes with an insight into the requirements and methods used in developing successful approaches for those experiencing alcohol-related problems. A deliberate attempt has been made to avoid the use of jargon, and where terminology has been used, to offer clear explanation and understanding.

The alcohol field holds many ambiguities, not least the use of the terms 'standard drink,' or 'units of alcohol.' Chapter 2 'What is a "standard drink"?' explains the difficulties experienced by researchers in the use of this term and thus this will not be developed further here. Clarity, and one's understanding, is not helped by the fact that 'one unit of alcohol,' implies the same as 'one standard drink'! Throughout this book, we have chosen to use the term 'standard drink', as the acceptable measure.

Specific gender is used as the author feels appropriate. However, unless stated, the use of the male/female gender is interchangeable. That is, we acknowledge that nurses can be male and patients or clients can be female.

Alcohol Use is intended as a resource for those – student or professional – new to the speciality of alcohol use and who wish to become specialist practitioners, or to update or refresh existing knowledge, or to develop services for this client group.

The analogy of the house purchaser perhaps best sums up the approach of the editor and authors when writing this book. Once the individual has identified a need to find out more about a property, the first step is to visit the potential house of purchase. On arrival, the potential purchaser obtains a quick view of the surrounding area, the look of the outside of the house and the open front door. This provides the basis for a decision to be made as to whether sufficient is known about the property or if more information is needed on which to base a decision to proceed or withdraw. This book takes the reader to the front door of alcohol use. It offers the basics. For some, that is all that will be needed: a point where sufficient information has been accessed so that the individual can then decide at what stage more information or guidance is needed on some of the many and diverse directions one can take working within the alcohol field.

As with any house purchase, as the potential purchaser passes the front door and enters each room, more is learnt about the property, the people who live there and those who surround the house. If the purchaser buys the property then more knowledge about the house, perfections and imperfections, will be gained. New things will be found out, some repairs made, some replacements, and new directions taken. The same applies to working with alcohol use and its related problems. One can never know all there is to know. There is a need to remain open minded in the individual approach to individual identified need. It is essential to be holistic and eclectic when accessing new information and knowledge. This applies both in terms of self-learning, and the way the professional approaches interventions with those who are in need of advice and guidance in their interactions with alcohol use and associated problems.

Each chapter provides direction to further learning and exploration. The book will not make the reader an expert. There is no such thing. The field is too broad. However, many learned professionals are willing to share their knowledge, and listen to the knowledge and advice of others. It is hoped that this basic introduction to alcohol use will stimulate the reader to open more doors to those in need of therapeutic interventions resultant from a problem related to their own or someone else's alcohol use.

PART ONE

General and epidemiological issues

What is a 'standard drink'?[a]

Marjana Martinic

Background

The practice of standardising drinks has long been implemented in commercial settings in which alcohol is available. Drink measures poured in licensed premises are used to standardise the volume of a given beverage sold to patrons and are controlled by licensing authorities. Commercial measures of most forms of beverage alcohol often vary from one country to another and are largely shaped by local drinking customs. In many European countries, for example, wine is served in decilitre increments and the British pint and half-pint are the staple servings of draught beer in pubs. Serving sizes of spirits are also often standardised in most industrialised countries.

From the public health perspective, the concept of a 'standard drink' was introduced as a means of advising the public whether they are drinking within reasonable thresholds for avoiding potential harm and whether they are likely to experience the health benefits of alcohol. Since then, the standard drink has been a central feature in some alcohol education campaigns, predominantly in English-speaking countries,[1] and has been used as a practical way of implementing government recommendations and guidelines on drinking. A 'safe' or 'low risk' number of standard drinks is based largely on existing medical evidence on long-term harm associated with different drinking levels and was designed as a tool to aid the public in avoiding potential harm.

While the premise underlying the standard drink is straightforward, the manner in which standard drinks are applied can be confusing. International comparisons are made difficult by a wide range of definitions. This disparity is often not taken into consideration when information on drinking guidelines from different countries, often given in terms of standard drinks or units, is interpreted and compared. The lack of a uniformly accepted standard measure also creates some difficulty for the purposes of research.

International definitions of a standard drink

The term 'standard drink' was originally intended to apply to drinks of 'standard' strengths. In practice, alcohol content varies among different beers, wines and distilled spirits. In addition, interpretations differ across countries of how much alcohol is contained in one standard drink. As Figure 2.1 illustrates, the range of official government definitions of standard drinks is wide.[2] The measure of unit sizes ranges from the equivalent of 8 grams of ethanol in the United Kingdom to 19.75 grams of ethanol in a Japanese standard drink, or *go*.[3]

Standard serving sizes may also differ within a given country depending on the type of beverage being served, so that the amount of alcohol contained in a serving of beer may be different from the amount in a serving of wine or of distilled spirits.[b] In Austria, for instance, a *Trinkeinheit*, or drink unit, is the equivalent of 12 grams of ethanol for beer or wine, or 6 grams of ethanol for spirits. These definitions are largely dependent on the accepted and prevailing practices in different countries. According to a report from China, in early 1997 the Beijing Technology Supervision Bureau introduced the litre as a standard measure for beer.[4] For full strength beer, this volume equals approximately 40 grams of ethanol. In the beerhalls of Zimbabwe, a standard serving mug contains 2 litres of beer,[5] often shared by several people. In the United States, standard-serving sizes of beer (12 oz), wine

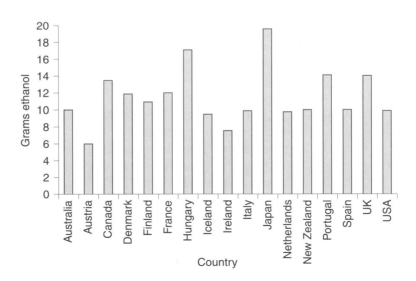

Figure 2.1 Official government definitions of a 'standard drink'.

(5 oz) and spirits (1.5 oz) are all officially defined as containing the equivalent of 14 grams of ethanol.[6]

The lack of uniformity in the definition of the standard drink is compounded by cultural preferences for the way in which alcohol content is measured – grams versus ounces of ethanol, American versus British fluid ounces, or measures of alcohol content as a percentage by weight or by volume. While official definitions of standard drinks may exist, the sizes of drinks poured in serving establishments often do not conform to them. A significant amount of beverage alcohol consumption occurs in homes and other private settings where drinks are rarely measured in standard units. These wide discrepancies and variations make any form of international comparison of drinks and consumption data difficult.

Some countries have attempted to introduce measures that would allow a better estimate of the number of standard drinks in a container of beverage alcohol. In Australia, a standard drink labelling of containers is required. In the United Kingdom, several beverage alcohol producers have recently made a voluntary decision to specify the number of UK units in a container of beverage alcohol on its label.

A drink is a drink – or is it?

Standard drinks are useful for the implementation of drinking guidelines and for the dissemination of messages to the general population. However, they are also used as a research tool for quantifying drinking levels and for describing the drinking patterns of individuals. Given the need for comparisons and applicability of data across countries, researchers report the lack of a uniform standard drink as particularly problematic within the research setting.

Units used by researchers often correspond to the standards accepted in their respective countries. However, not all researchers adhere to government-issued standards when analysing their data, but rather derive their own definitions from different sources. This lack of uniformity results in further confusion. A study undertaken by Turner illustrates this problem.[7] This comparison of definitions of standard drinks used in 125 international epidemiological studies showed that the definitions of a 'drink' ranged from 8 grams of ethanol in the United Kingdom to 28 grams of ethanol in some Japanese studies.

When the standard drink approach is applied to the assessment of harm, the problem of definitions is amplified still further. In the epidemiological literature, drinking behaviours and drinking levels at which problems may occur are often defined in terms of particular numbers of drinks. For instance, by some North American definitions, a 'binge' is defined as five or more drinks in a row for males.[8,9] Similarly, the benchmark for 'harmful' drinking is sometimes set at nine or more drinks in a row.[10]

The problem becomes clear when one compares what these definitions of a 'binge' or of 'harmful' drinking mean when different interpretations of a 'drink' are applied, as illustrated in Figure 2.2.[c] Using the five-drink definition, a 'binge' would amount to the equivalent of 40 grams of absolute ethanol in Ireland; in Hungary, on the other hand, it would equal 85 grams of ethanol, or more than twice that amount. Similarly, the nine or more drinks definition for harmful drinking would mean that a Japanese drinker would have to consume the equivalent of 178 grams of absolute ethanol to qualify. An Austrian, on the other hand, could reach this point after 54 grams.

Much of the data used for the assessment of harm are collected through surveys. Respondents are asked to report on their levels of drinking in terms of the number of drinks they have consumed. These self-reported values are then standardised by researchers into drink or ethanol equivalents. Whether these standardised values can accurately be used for research purposes is a complicated issue. Data derived from self-report questionnaires rely heavily on the ability of respondents to remember the number of drinks they have consumed within a given period of time, which can cover a day, a week, months, or even a year.

The reliability of this method is further compromised by the lack of uniform definitions used by either governments or researchers. There is also the additional problem that survey respondents are required to recall the amount of alcohol they have consumed and report it as a given

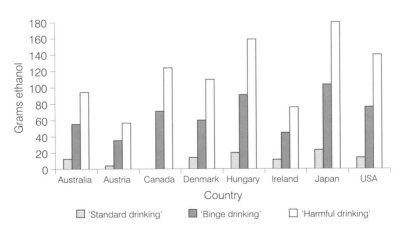

Figure 2.2 Official government definitions of a 'standard drink', 'binge' and 'harmful drinking'.

number of drinks. The size of each drink must be estimated, taking into account both the alcohol content of the drink and the size of the container. Both of these variables are difficult to gauge. As a study by Stockwell and Stirling has shown, most people are unable to estimate the size or strength of a drink with accuracy.[11] The degree of accuracy decreases even further when the alcohol content of the beverage is either lower or higher than average. As another study has suggested, the deviation appears to be highest for distilled spirits and lowest for wine.[12]

In some countries, glasses in which wine, beer or spirits are served in many establishments are marked at a particular level so that the amount of alcohol consumed can be gauged. In other countries, such as the United States, standardised serving sizes are not required, meaning that the amount of alcohol in a particular drink can vary and is often larger than the government definition of a standard drink. Much drinking also occurs in off-premise settings in which drinks are generally not served in standard sizes or containers and partially filled glasses are often replenished, making an estimate of the number of drinks consumed difficult. In many developing countries, where drinking is a communal activity and drinks are often consumed from a common container, any attempt to quantify numbers of drinks may be a hopeless one altogether.

Conclusions

As this report has attempted to illustrate, the way in which the concept of a standard drink is currently implemented within an international setting is less than optimal. For the purposes of research and for cross-cultural comparisons, the usefulness of the 'standard drink' hinges upon international consensus on the way in which it is defined. The challenge is to establish acceptable criteria for standardising units of measurement and to strive towards greater harmonisation in the way in which the concept of a standard drink is used. It has been suggested that a unit of measurement expressed in terms of grams of ethanol should be adopted to standardise 'standard drinks'.

At the same time, harmonisation of drink sizes is not necessarily a practical option when it comes to educating the public. Counting drinks for the purposes of epidemiology is not a common practice among most drinkers, and drink sizes used within countries are often reflections of the culture. The notion of 'standard drinks' may not be an easy one to reconcile with many accepted drinking practices. From the point of view of educating the public about sensible drinking, guidelines that are in keeping with local drinking practices and drinking cultures seem a more reasonable approach.

Notes

a This chapter was first published as *What is a 'Standard Drink'? Report 5*; September 1998, International Center for Alcohol Policies, Washington, DC, and is reproduced by kind permission of Professor Marcus Grant, President, ICAP and the author, Marjana Martinic, Director of Science Policy.

The International Center for Alcohol Policies (ICAP) is dedicated to helping reduce the abuse of alcohol worldwide and to promoting understanding of the role of alcohol in society through dialogue and partnerships involving the beverage alcohol industry, the public heath community and others interested in alcohol policy. ICAP is a not-for-profit organisation supported by 10 major international beverage alcohol companies.

b The Austrian Bundesministerium fur Gesundheit und Konsumentenschutz defines standard drinks or *Trinkeinheiten* in a beverage-specific way. The measures used are 125 ml (approximately 12 g ethanol) of wine, 300 ml (approximately 12 g of ethanol) of beer and 20 ml (approximately 6 g of ethanol) of spirits.

c For the purposes of this comparison, a 'binge' is defined as five or more drinks, and 'harmful' drinking is defined as nine or more drinks.

CHAPTER 3

Its use in perspective

Douglas Cameron

Learning objectives

To understand:

- the basic pharmacological effects of alcohol
- that the psychological effects of alcohol are learned
- that making drinking pleasurable involves adjusting dose to setting and purpose
- that there are wide variations in acceptable drinking styles
- that people also vary greatly within any culture as to how central drinking is to their way of life
- how people may become designated as problematic drinkers.

The substance

At room temperature, alcohol (specifically ethyl alcohol, ethanol) is a clear, unpleasant-smelling, raw-tasting liquid. Humans consume it by mouth because they have learned that it can engender changes in their mental states: their moods, their levels of relaxation and their sociability. It is not consumed 'neat', but is consumed diluted with water and has added to it a wide variety of flavourings, the majority of which occur naturally as part of the production process. Alcoholic beverages come in a variety of tastes and with differing concentrations of alcohol in them.

Pharmacologically, alcohol is a basal narcotic, a central nervous system depressant which affects all brain areas, including those concerned with our most fundamental life functions: breathing, staying awake, responding to the world around us. If the dose ingested is very high, alcohol acts like a general anaesthetic: it renders the consumer unconscious. If the dose is low, the body, particularly the liver, breaks down and disposes of the substance sufficiently quickly for the consumer to be unaware or hardly aware of having ingested it. People have to consume alcohol of sufficient concentration at a sufficient rate to induce the effects that they have learned to expect from it. For this to happen, the blood alcohol level has to rise at a rate somewhere between the two rates shown in Figure 3.1.

As it happens, the amount of pure (absolute) alcohol dispensed per glass in social situations is broadly the same, regardless of the beverage. One glass of table wine, one smaller glass of fortified wine (port, sherry or vermouth), a single 'pub' measure of spirits and one half-pint of ordinary strength beer all contain approximately what has latterly become known in Britain as a standard unit (sometimes referred to as a 'standard drink' – see Chapter 2), 8 grams or 10 millilitres of absolute alcohol (Box 3.1).[a] This helps consumers to maintain their blood alcohol level in the required range and of course was the practice long before the recent popularisation of 'counting standard drinks'.

Box 3.1 Standard drinks of alcohol

The amount of alcohol in these drinks is approximately the same (8.0 grams or 10.0 millilitres):

- one glass of table wine
- one glass of fortified wine (port, sherry, vermouth)
- one single measure of spirits
- one half-pint of ordinary strength beer.

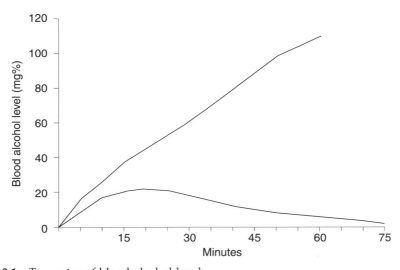

Figure 3.1 Two rates of blood alcohol levels.

Whilst the effects of alcohol do depend in part on the overall level of alcohol in the body, they are also dependent upon rate of change of those levels. In the same way as we notice not only the speed we travel in our cars but also whether we are accelerating or decelerating, so we notice whether our blood alcohol level is rising or falling. A falling blood alcohol level induces rather different feelings from a rising one. This is called the Mellanby effect, after the pharmacologist who first described it. If a rising curve makes a drinker relaxed, talkative and sociable, the falling curve is likely to induce the opposite: irritability and withdrawal. To avoid these feelings, consumers carefully titrate their blood alcohol levels to rise steadily during a drinking session, and normally undertake such sessions in the evening so that they can be asleep as the alcohol is being broken down and eliminated from the body and the blood alcohol level is falling.

Clearly, getting the most out of alcohol requires considerable skill on the part of the consumer and that skill has to be acquired over time. The task of learning to drink is never over. Adults are perpetually adjusting their drinking styles to changing situations. Whilst it might be acceptable for a young, football-playing male to get thoroughly intoxicated with his mates after the Saturday afternoon match and to have a hangover on Sunday morning, it might be quite unacceptable for that same man some years later to get intoxicated to that same degree, with that same consequence, when staying for the weekend with the boss!

Intoxication

Although alcohol is a very simple molecule, its effects are far from simple. It affects cell membranes, hence ion transfer in and out of cells and a wide range of neurotransmitters. The mental effects are similarly complex. The effects that alcohol has on an individual consumer depend upon many factors:

- the person doing the consuming
- the mood they were in before they started consuming
- the expectancies they bring with them into the drinking occasion
- the intent
- the site of consumption
- the company or lack of it
- the behaviour of those surrounding the drinker
- the time of day.

We have known for more than 30 years, and certainly since the appearance of a landmark book by McAndrew and Edgerton in 1969,

Drunken Comportment,[1] that the conventional wisdom about alcohol – that it is a depressant which disinhibits by suppression of the controlling effects exerted by the higher brain centres – is a gross oversimplification. What seems to occur is disinhibition *within limits*.

The arguments these authors make for this are threefold:

1 there are societies whose members' drunken comportment fails to exhibit anything 'disinhibited'
2 drunken comportment varies over historical time
3 drunken comportment varies radically from one set of socially ordered situations or circumstances to another.

What this means is that the experience of drunkenness and behaviours allowable when in that state are socially determined and learned:

• if we learn that alcohol relaxes us, so it does
• if we learn that alcohol induces belligerence or rowdiness, so it does.

In psychological jargon, alcohol intoxication is a *discriminative stimulus* for the release of a range of social (or, indeed, antisocial) behaviours.

It is also important to note that the word 'drunk' has a number of meanings. McKechnie[2] defined 'drunkenness' in four ways:

1 the emotional state produced by any level of alcoholisation
2 the emotional state produced by extreme degrees of alcoholisation
3 the behaviour produced by extreme degrees of alcoholisation
4 a retrospective definition based on subsequent events: 'I must have been drunk because … I've got a hangover, I don't remember what happened … I fell over on the dance floor …'.[2]

These definitions are interesting for they do not carry positive or negative connotations. It may or may not be useful to the individual to be in that state. These definitions do not convey that to be drunk is socially desirable or undesirable. To be drunk is simply to be in a particular state induced by the ingestion of alcohol.

Self-assessment questions: thinking about drinking

Ask yourself the following questions:

1 The last time you had a drink:

- How much did you consume?
- Where did you drink?
- With whom did you drink?
- What was the purpose of your drinking?

2 The time before that:

- How much did you consume?
- Where did you drink?
- With whom did you drink?
- What was the purpose of your drinking?

3 Were those two drinking events the same? If not, what were the differences?

Drinking styles

People drink in different ways for different reasons on different occasions. Accomplished drinkers have a number of drinking styles. They use intoxication for different purposes on different occasions. An individual drinking occasion has a spectrum of different meanings from external to internal. A drinking event with external meaning, for instance, would be drinking at a family wedding to celebrate the occasion. One with internal meaning would be, say, 'to drown one's sorrows' or to have 'time out'. That is functional drinking. Between these two there is a general category which has been called subcultural. A subcultural drinking style is one where engaging in a drinking event is in part functional, for personal effect, but also in part because it is a way of life, e.g. going to the pub to meet friends after work on Friday night. Therefore, this dimension can be divided into three broad categories:

1 occasional
2 subcultural
3 functional.

There is clearly a relationship between the purpose and meaning of a drinking event and the dose of alcohol consumed. If the meaning of a drinking event is escape, then higher doses are more likely to be useful. Conversely, to have a high dose of alcohol at an occasional event, such as a Roman Catholic or Anglican Christian communion service, is quite unacceptable. Thus there is a two-dimensional matrix between dose and meaning of a drinking event. This is shown in Figure 3.2.

		Dose		
		Low	*Intermediate*	*High*
Meaning	*Occasional*			
	Subcultural			
	Functional			

Figure 3.2 Two-dimensional matrix between dose and meaning of drink.

As well as dose and meaning on any particular drinking occasion, there is also the issue of setting or site of drinking, where the drinking takes place. To get drinking right on any single attempt, it is necessary to understand three things:

1 the meaning (or purpose)
2 the dose
3 the site.

McKechnie[3] has drawn this out (Figure 3.3). If, as in column 1, all three are right, the drinking is *appropriate*. In column 2, there is an error of dosage. The purpose or meaning might be socialising on a special occasion, say a family wedding. The site is right – the reception. However, one drinker drinks so much that he falls asleep in the corner of the room – an error of overdosage. An example of a column 3 error would be for a drinker to be drinking functionally, perhaps to be going for oblivion when others in the company are subculturally drinking – for conviviality. The single drinker may behave in a sullen, antisocial way. A column 4 error could be, for example, convivial drinking of moderate doses with friends but in the wrong place, such as upstairs in a bus on the way home from work.

	1	2	3	4	5	6	7	8
Dose	✓	X	✓	✓	✓	X	X	X
Purpose	✓	✓	X	✓	X	✓	X	X
Site	✓	✓	✓	X	X	X	✓	X

Figure 3.3   McKechnie's Grid – issues related to setting, site or purpose of drinking.[3]

Getting all three conditions right is not easy and most drinkers get it wrong on occasion and learn from their errors. That is the process by which people never stop learning to drink: constant adjustments to drinking styles take place.

Theoretically, all eight styles in the dose/meaning matrix can occur, but obviously some are more common than others. Kilty[4] explored some American drinking styles and used a cluster analysis of data from questionnaire-based interviews to analyse the answers. This involves looking at all the answers and noting which ones are identical or similar to each other – which seem to belong together – to form a cluster. He found that four of the clusters – the styles – reported by his subjects accounted for two-thirds of the variance. He called them factors and they are shown in Box 3.2.

Box 3.2 Drinking styles[4]

Factor 1: Convivial drinking (24.5%)
Factor 2: Thirst quenching (18.3%)
Factor 3: Alcohol and lifestyle (14.1%)
Factor 4: Changing one's mood (9.6%)

These styles can be readily, but not perfectly, fitted onto the dose/meaning matrix (see Figure 3.2). Convivial drinking is likely to be occasional or subcultural and low or intermediate dose; thirst quenching: functional, low dose; alcohol and lifestyle: subcultural, any dose; and changing one's mood: functional, any dose.

Drinker types

This chapter has so far discussed only the single drinking *event*, or session. There is another dimension of drinking which is clearly relevant, and that concerns the *drinkers*. It is about how important it is to an individual to engage in these drinking events, about how central drinking is to that person. Drinking can be on a spectrum from irrelevant to a person's life, quite peripheral to utterly central to their everyday existence. Most drinkers are intermediately placed between these two extremes. So, there are now three dimensions of a drinker relating to how important the drinking of alcohol is to them in pursuing the kind of drinking style. This is shown in Box 3.3.

Box 3.3 Dimensions of a drinker

DOSE
Low – Intermediate – High

MEANING
Occasional – Subcultural – Functional

CENTRALITY
Peripheral – Intermediate – Central

That gives us a 3 × 3 × 3 matrix of 27 possible positions, like a Rubik's cube. Theoretically, there can be 27 different drinker types from, at one corner, a low-dose, special occasion drinker for whom drinking is peripheral to their everyday lives to, in the opposite corner, a high-dose, functional drinker for whom being intoxicated *is* their life. In addition, of course, there are many possible permutations between those two extremes. For instance, a high-dose occasional and peripheral drinker might be a Scot who gets drunk only at Hogmanay.

Adding this third dimension changes our perspective from drinking styles to drinker types and in the same piece of work mentioned above, Kilty[4] has empirically derived a typology of them.

Again, it is possible to fit these drinker types onto the theoretical 3 × 3 × 3 matrix (Box 3.4):

- type 1 includes those nine types who are functional drinkers, of all centralities and doses, one complete side of the Rubik's cube
- type 2 are occasional, low-dose and peripheral drinkers
- type 3 are functional, low-dose peripherals. Then we see some gender differences
- types 4 and 5 are both intermediate-dose, subcultural and either intermediate or fully central drinkers, but the men drink beer and the women drink a variety of beverages as an expression of lifestyle

---

Box 3.4 Drinker types[4]

1   Drinkers who use alcohol to alter their moods
2   Light drinkers who dislike the taste of alcohol
3   Light drinkers who use alcohol as an occasional thirst-quencher
4   New middle-class male beer drinkers
5   New sophisticated middle-class women drinkers
6   Moderate social drinkers.

Lastly,

• type 6 drinkers are intermediate-dose subcultural drinkers for whom drinking can be anywhere on the centrality dimension.

It is important to recognise that just as drinking styles are not fixed for an individual, a drinker adapts her or his drinking style to the circumstances in which they choose to go drinking, so drinker types are not permanent either. As their lifestyles, incomes and social circumstances change, people move from being one type of drinker to another. Drinking becomes less central in a young male drinker's life depending, typically, upon whether they have met up with a partner with whom they want to set up home. Even people whose drinking has brought them to the attention of treatment agencies may, with suitable guidance and support, be able to change from the type of drinker they were at presentation to become, or become again, a predominantly subcultural low-dose drinker with their drinking no longer central to their lives.[5]

Problematic drinking?

It is now worthwhile to look at where so-called problem drinkers occur within this theoretical matrix. Largely, the definition of what is problem drinking is socially determined. What is deemed problematic in one culture or subculture is not so labelled in another.

One example of how a culture defines its problem drinkers was provided by Mulford.[6] He examined the community labelling process in Iowa, USA, and found two drinking styles, one drinker type and one drinking consequence which, if displayed by a drinker, made it more likely that such a person would be labelled a problem drinker. These four phenomena were cumulative and non-sequential. The more of these four 'stigmata' one demonstrated, the more likely one was to be labelled a problem drinker or 'alcoholic'.

Using our theoretical $3 \times 3 \times 3$ matrix again, Mulford's (Box 3.5) factor 1, trouble due to drinking, can occur in any of the 27 drinker types if they get dose, purpose or setting wrong, as illustrated in McKechnie's matrix (see Figure 3.3). However, an individual whose drinking is functional (Mulford's factor 2), whose drinking is central (Mulford's factor 3), and who tends to drink large doses (Mulford's factor 4) is much more liable, in Iowa, to be labelled as a problem drinker.

Box 3.5 Factors in community labelling[6]

1 Trouble due to drinking
2 Personal effect drinking
3 Preoccupied drinking
4 Uncontrolled drinking.

It is worth underlining that according to the people of Iowa, and it is unlikely that they are unusual, it is those people for whom drinking is personally effective and who drink frequently because of that who are in danger of having their drinking labelled as problematic. Conversely, those who drink a little because of the social circumstances in which they find themselves, who respond to 'peer pressure', but are not seeking or achieving any worthwhile psychological effects and who may well not really like what they are doing are most unlikely to be called problem drinkers. Drinking appears to be yet another behaviour, in which we can engage, but only if we feel pressurised into it and do not enjoy it!

The important thing about examining drinking in the essentially theoretical way that has been done in this chapter is that it is a way of looking at the phenomena of drinkers and drinking *without* getting involved in the kind of moral issues which crept into the last paragraph. The language used to describe drinkers-who-break-the-rules has varied over time: habitual drunkard, chronic inebriate, alcoholic, alcohol addict, sufferer from the alcohol dependence syndrome and problem drinker. The phenomena that these drinkers display to be so labelled are not fixed, either within a culture or over time.

To develop your knowledge in this area, see 'To learn more', p. 248.

Note

a On mainland Europe, the standard drink is one-fifth larger, being 10.0 grams of absolute alcohol.

Self-assessment questions

1 What volume of alcohol does a British 'standard unit' contain?
2 List some factors that determine the psychological effects of alcohol.
3 What does *drunk* mean?
4 What is functional drinking?
5 What factors make it likely that a drinker will be labelled problematic?

CHAPTER 4

The body and its health

Alex Paton

Pre-reading exercise

On Figure 4.1, label the parts of the body you feel will be affected by inappropriate or excessive alcohol use. When you have read the chapter, repeat the exercise to see if your understanding is the same or has improved. You can check this on p. 228, Chapter 4 answers. This exercise should take about 15 minutes to complete.

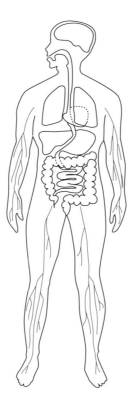

Figure 4.1 Body diagram.[a]

Summary

- Knowledge of the way in which alcohol is handled by the body provides a basis for understanding its beneficial effects in small quantities and the harm caused by excessive drinking.
- Absorption from the stomach, distribution through the body and breakdown (metabolism) by liver enzymes are determined by physiological and biochemical mechanisms; these are subject to gender differences, genetic influences, environmental pressures and the experience of drinking.
- The liver has a large reserve of dehydrogenase enzymes which can deal with considerable quantities of alcohol by oxidation to acetaldehyde and then to harmless acetate which enters the normal metabolic pool.
- Excessive production of acetaldehyde, a highly toxic substance, or different types of dehydrogenase might explain why certain individuals are liable to be damaged, but evidence so far is contradictory.
- Compared with psychosocial harm, physical damage from excessive drinking is uncommon, though almost every bodily organ is vulnerable.
- Most people in Britain drink within sensible limits, a minority drink heavily and a few become addicted to alcohol (dependent) or are physically damaged, usually irreversibly. Because it is not yet possible to predict who will be damaged, early detection of those suffering physical problems is essential.
- Three types of physical damage can be distinguished:
- acute effects, from intoxication and binge drinking, resulting in accidents, cerebral damage and serious metabolic disturbances
- features of ill health, particularly affecting the gastrointestinal tract, heart and nervous system, which because they are non-specific may not be recognised as due to heavy drinking
- diseases like cirrhosis, cardiomyopathy and brain syndromes which are relatively uncommon and affect a minority of the heaviest drinkers for reasons which are unknown.

Alcohol (C_2H_5OH, ethyl alcohol, ethanol) is a drug.[b] It is unlikely to have been approved for use if it had been introduced today, yet its value as a social, religious and medicinal lubricant has been apparent since the birth of civilisation. 'In the beginning there was alcohol',[1] and such is 'man's [and increasingly woman's] insatiable thirst for a pleasant poison'[2] that few cultures survive without it, and only Islam, among the major religions, prohibits its use.

Cultural and religious attitudes are only two of the many determinants of drinking; they are part of a complex of behavioural and environmental factors (nurture) which include age, sex, psychosocial functioning, family drinking patterns, social and peer pressures, affluence and availability of drink. It is possible that genetic factors (nature) may be involved because genes influence enzymes concerned in the metabolism of alcohol (see later) as well as chemical neurotransmitters in the brain, but they play only a minor part, perhaps up to a third, in most heavy drinking.[3]

Alcohol acts as a sedative by altering neurotransmitter activity; it was once used as a rather inefficient anaesthetic. Moderate quantities (two to six standard drinks – see also Chapter 2) produce feelings of well-being, relaxation and mild euphoria, with loosening of inhibitions, hence its value in facilitating social intercourse. Even at these levels, judgement may be impaired and reaction times reduced, so that accidents are more likely. Intoxication from continued drinking produces physical and mental changes (Table 4.1) that can be roughly predicted from the amount drunk and breath or blood alcohol concentrations (BAC). Women and young drinkers become intoxicated at lower BACs than men because they are more sensitive to equivalent doses of alcohol, while hardened drinkers may not show symptoms even at very high BACs through development of tolerance (p. 30).

Table 4.1 Physical and mental effects at different blood alcohol concentrations

Blood alcohol concentration mg/100 ml	Effects
30	Disinhibition, mild euphoria
50	Impairment of skills and judgement
80	Motor impairment
	Accident risk doubled
100	Garrulous, elated, aggressive
160	**Accident risk increased tenfold**
200	Slurred speech, gross unsteadiness
400	Coma Death from respiratory failure or inhalation of vomit

A variety of physiological effects accompany drinking:

- stimulation of the circulation causes flushing, sweating and tachycardia
- the pituitary and adrenal glands release increased amounts of stress hormones

- the gonads produce more sex hormones
- the kidneys secrete more urine, not only because of the quantities of fluid drunk but also because their own hormones are activated.

Most people enjoy modest drinking, a minority consistently drink over the odds, and an even smaller number become dependent or are physically damaged (Table 4.2). The more a *population* drinks (per capita consumption) the greater the number of *individuals* harmed. Serious physical damage, however, is infrequent, involving perhaps fewer than 10% of heavy drinkers, and is numerically insignificant compared with the considerable burden of psychological, socio-economic and legal problems.

Table 4.2 Definition of drinking patterns (these figures are approximate guidelines)

Drinking pattern		Units per week
Social	– within normal limits	men 21
		women 14
Moderate	– occasional drinking over limits	
Heavy	– hazardous: socio-economic and minor physical problems	men 22–29
		women 15–35
	– harmful: risk of physical damage	men >50
		women >36
Binge (on any one occasion)		men 10 +
		women 7 +
Dependent – drink takes over life		men >50
		women >36

Alcohol in the body

Alcohol is a small molecule that is rapidly absorbed from the stomach and upper part of the small intestine and diffuses readily throughout the body. Rate of absorption is most rapid when the stomach is empty, and when the concentration of alcohol is between 20–30%. Thus sherry (30%) raises the BAC more rapidly than beer (3–8%), while neat spirits (40%) delay gastric emptying and have an inhibitory effect on alcohol absorption. Food, particularly starches and fats, also delays absorption. The best way to take alcohol is with meals, or in the case of spirits, with some form of diluent.

Over 90% of alcohol is extracted from the blood and is widely distributed in body water, so that vital organs like brain, heart and muscles are exposed to the same concentration as in the blood. The liver is particularly vulnerable because it receives blood direct from the stomach and intestines via the portal system. Fat is a poor absorber of alcohol because it has little blood supply; this may partly explain why women, with more subcutaneous fat and a smaller blood volume than men, achieve a higher BAC for a given amount of alcohol. They also have lower levels of alcohol dehydrogenases (see below) in the stomach, so that more alcohol is absorbed. BAC is also dependent on size, body build, previous exposure to alcohol and drug use; it varies with the menstrual cycle in women, being highest in the premenstrual and ovulatory phases.[4]

About 15 mg of alcohol (two standard drinks) are cleared from 100 ml blood per hour, and the liver breaks down about one standard drink an hour, so that it is possible to calculate the likely peak BAC and rate of clearance after given amounts of alcohol (Table 4.3).

Table 4.3 Peak alcohol concentration and clearance after various amounts (standard drinks) of alcohol

Standard drinks (or units) of alcohol	Peak blood alcohol concentration mg/100ml	Clearance hours
3	50	3
6	100	6
10	200	13

Alcohol is largely metabolised (broken down) by enzymes in the liver; only 2–5% is excreted unchanged in the urine, sweat and breath. The first step is oxidation of alcohol to acetaldehyde by alcohol dehydrogenases (ADH). Acetaldehyde is a highly reactive and toxic substance, which has been suspected of causing physical damage, but it is rapidly converted by acetaldehyde dehydrogenases (ALDH) to harmless acetate (Figure 4.2).

When the liver has to deal with large amounts of alcohol, a number of chemical products accumulate which can have clinical consequences:

- *lactate* can disturb acid base balance
- *urate* causes gout
- *glucose* may aggravate diabetes
- *triglycerides* (fats) give a milky appearance to the blood and accumulate in muscle and liver.

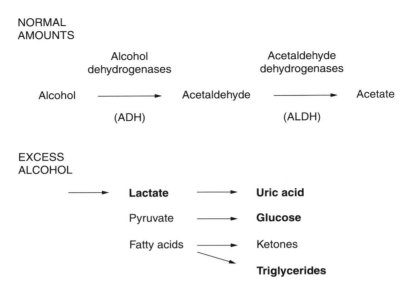

Figure 4.2 Metabolism of alcohol. Harmful products are indicated in bold type.

Persistent heavy drinkers are able to metabolise greater than normal amounts of alcohol ('tolerance') because of 'enzyme induction', by which production of ADH is greatly increased and other enzymes are stimulated to help dispose of the alcohol.

Physical effects

Alcohol can affect most bodily organs, so that heavy drinkers are liable to suffer from many types of ill health (Box 4.1); it is important to recognise these for what they are[5] because intervention can prevent progression to serious disease. The rarer classical diseases, like cirrhosis and brain damage, are the result of years of drinking, and when they come to medical attention the outlook is often poor – so-called 'end stage disease'. At least 33 000 deaths a year in England and Wales are currently attributed to alcohol;[6] they are likely to be premature, in 40–50-year-olds, and women die earlier than men. So many diseases have been ascribed to alcohol that only the most important can be discussed here.

Box 4.1 Physical pointers to heavy drinking

- Gastrointestinal tract – anorexia, heartburn, morning sickness, gastritis, dyspepsia, diarrhoea
- Heart – chest pain (sometimes mimicking angina), palpitations
- Recurrent chest infections
- Repeated accidents
- Tendency to bleeding – bruises, gums, nose
- Absence from work due to 'illness', especially after weekend (Monday morning syndrome)
- Psychological problems – headaches, inability to concentrate, insomnia, anxiety, 'depression'
- Menstrual irregularities, sexual problems, infertility
- In the elderly: confusion, falls, incontinence, hypothermia

Heart and circulation

Perhaps the best known (and certainly best advertised) association of alcohol with the heart is its protective effect against death from *ischaemic (coronary) heart disease* (IHD). This occurs with as little as one to two standard drinks of alcohol two or three times a week, and is thought to be due to reduction in clotting and a rise in levels of protective lipoproteins, thus delaying atheroma in the coronary arteries. Death rates are particularly low in wine-drinking countries, hence the suggestion that wine should be drunk, but the current belief is that alcohol itself is the protective factor.[7] The benefit of larger amounts of alcohol is controversial; heavy drinking *increases* the risks, particularly of sudden death from myocardial infarction, and of course may damage other organs.

A rarer type of heart disease is *cardiomyopathy*, in which the heart muscle is damaged by alcohol, with resultant heart failure. Formerly almost exclusive to men, it is now increasingly encountered in women. More uncommon is *beri-beri*, a type of acute heart failure due to lack of vitamin B_1 (thiamine), usually from beer drinking. It can be cured by giving thiamine, provided the individual stops drinking.

It is not always appreciated that alcohol can cause *arrhythmias* (disorders of the heartbeat), such as atrial fibrillation and ventricular tachycardias, by poisoning the conducting system of the heart. In America this is known as 'holiday heart' because it tends to occur in people who binge at weekends or on holiday, especially if they are unaccustomed to large quantities of alcohol. Arrhythmias can also develop in persistent heavy drinkers; they respond well to cutting down the drink. Ventricular fibrillation, though, is particularly dangerous and can cause sudden, unexpected death.

There is a positive relationship between blood pressure (BP) and the amount of alcohol drunk: in a population of drinkers the blood pressure begins to rise with as little as two standard drinks a day.[8] Alcohol has been found to be a significant cause of *hypertension* in up to 30% of patients,[9] particularly in men who drink six or more standard drinks a day; reducing drinking may normalise the blood pressure or at least reduce the amount of drugs needed to control it. About a quarter of drinkers undergoing detoxification have hypertension when first seen, which returns to normal after a few days of withdrawal (Figure 4.3), probably due to stimulation of hormones which control blood pressure.

Stomach and intestines

Heavy drinkers are prone to *oesophagitis* and sometimes bleeding due to a tear caused by vomiting (Mallory–Weiss syndrome), *gastritis* and failure to absorb nutrients from the intestine. It is debatable whether alcohol 'causes' gastric and duodenal ulcers but it certainly aggravates symptoms. People who drink 10 or more standard drinks a day run a risk (greater if

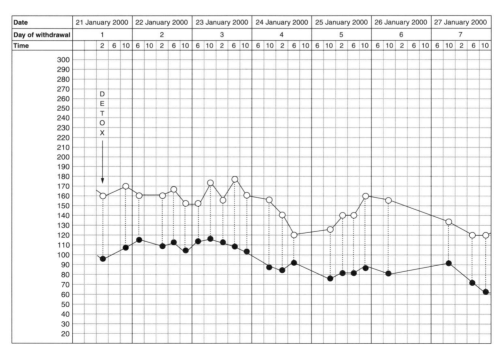

Figure 4.3 Blood pressure chart showing raised BP at start of detoxification, reducing as detoxification continues to the individual's normal BP.

they smoke as well) of *cancers of the aerodigestive tract* – mouth, oesophagus, pharynx and larynx.[10]

Chronic pancreatitis results from the destructive action of alcohol on the pancreas: repeated and extremely painful attacks of abdominal pain are followed by diarrhoea and failure to absorb nutrients (malabsorption) because of loss of pancreatic digestive juices, and eventually diabetes, when internal secretion of insulin fails.[11] To observe such an individual continuing to drink in spite of pain and wasting is to be reminded of the awesome grip of alcohol dependence.

Liver[12]

Liver disease is the best known physical effect of heavy drinking. Two pieces of evidence illustrate the causal connection: when wine was rationed in France during the Second World War there was a dramatic fall in deaths from cirrhosis; and a rising death rate accompanied increasing consumption of alcohol from the 1950s in all developed countries.

Most heavy drinkers have deposits of fat in the liver cells (*fatty liver*) because of difficulty in disposing of fatty acids. This is not thought to be a precursor of cirrhosis, and disappears with abstinence. Occasionally alcohol causes *hepatitis*, inflammation of the liver with jaundice (more common in women), which may progress to cirrhosis. Less than one in 10 persistent drinkers develops *cirrhosis*, in which the liver becomes progressively scarred by fibrous tissue which replaces liver cells. The risk of cirrhosis begins to rise with intakes of five standard drinks a day, but the average consumption of men with the disease is 20 standard drinks a day for at least eight years. Women are damaged by smaller quantities over shorter periods. Some 3000 deaths from alcoholic cirrhosis are reported in England and Wales each year,[6] but this figure is almost certainly an underestimate because of failure to record alcohol on the death certificate.

Because of its numerous biochemical functions, the liver is rich in enzymes. When the liver is stressed or damaged, enzymes leak from the cells into the bloodstream and can be measured to indicate the extent of damage. Gamma glutamyl transferase (GGT) is the most commonly used test in drinkers: values above 40 units per litre suggest moderate or heavy drinking, but it is important to bear in mind that like all biological tests they are only positive in some 70–80% of individuals. Aspartate aminotransferase (AST) and alanine aminotransferase (ALT) are more specifically related to serious liver damage: levels above 35 and 40 units per litre respectively suggest either heavy drinking or cirrhosis. The ratio of AST to ALT is said to be higher in alcoholic cirrhosis than in other types of liver damage.[13]

Brain and nervous system[14]

Alcohol excess can cause blackouts and amnesia, with sometimes fugue-like states in which individuals have no subsequent knowledge of their behaviour. *Seizures (fits)* may occur during acute intoxication or in heavy drinkers; they may also be encountered in alcohol withdrawal.[15] *Stroke*, especially in younger people and possibly related to hypertension,[16] *subarachnoid haemorrhage* and *subdural haematoma* after head injury are other complications.

A number of people who drink heavily develop cognitive impairment. Brain scanning even in young drinkers has shown loss of brain tissue and enlargement of ventricles,[17] and alcohol has been claimed as a common cause of *presenile dementia*. The features do not differ from those of other types of dementia: memory loss, cognitive impairment, emotional instability and personality changes result in slow deterioration over many years. Parkinson's disease may sometimes be alcohol related.

Withdrawal symptoms result from suddenly stopping alcohol or from stresses like infections, accidents and operations in individuals who are dependent on alcohol. Tremor, agitation, confusion, nausea, insomnia and auditory hallucinations are the usual features; sweating, tachycardia, hypertension and fever may also be present. A more serious form, seen in less than 10% of individuals, is *delirium tremens*, in which confusion and visual hallucinations, either fearful or amusing, supervene.[18]

Two rare, overlapping brain syndromes are associated with prolonged alcohol use; both are associated with thiamine deficiency from the combination of alcohol and defective diet.[19] *Wernicke's encephalopathy* is an acute condition caused by multiple, small haemorrhages in different parts of the brain resulting in a characteristic triad of abnormal eye movements, unsteadiness and a confusional state. *Korsakoff's syndrome* is characterised by apathy, confusion, disorientation and loss of memory for recent events, which results in confabulation and lack of insight. Prompt administration of thiamine by injection in the first instance arrests the acute features, but many patients are left with the memory disturbances of Korsakoff's syndrome which do not respond to thiamine.

Peripheral neuropathy (neuritis) – pins and needles, numbness and burning discomfort in the legs, sometimes with difficulty in walking – occurs more frequently in women than men. Thought to be due to a combination of thiamine deficiency and a direct toxic effect of alcohol, slow improvement over many months may follow abstinence but not by administration of thiamine alone.

Endocrine glands

The adrenal glands, which secrete cortisone, can be stimulated by alcohol. This sometimes causes *pseudo-Cushing's syndrome,* which mimics the condition caused by overactivity or tumours of the adrenal glands.[20] The characteristic features, seen in about one in five heavy drinkers, are a rounded, plethoric facies, obesity and hypertension. If alcohol is not recognised as the cause, patients may be subjected to unnecessary investigation; abstinence will reverse the condition.

A precipitate fall in blood sugar (*hypoglycaemia*) may follow a binge or drinking on an empty stomach, when liver glycogen that produces glucose is depleted. Excessive drowsiness or unruly behaviour should raise suspicions. Hypoglycaemia can be particularly dangerous in young children who consume alcohol because of their limited stores of glycogen.[21]

Reproductive system[22]

Heavy drinking by men may cause loss of libido and reduced potency; the testes shrink, sperm production is reduced and testosterone levels fall while oestrogens increase, resulting in 'feminisation' with loss of body hair and breast enlargement. These changes are most prominent in cirrhosis, but alcohol itself impairs male fertility; one study showed that reduced sperm production resulted from as little as four to six standard drinks of alcohol daily, and that this was improved in half the men after three months' abstinence.[23]

Women suffer from menstrual irregularities; fertility is reduced because alcohol affects the ovaries and reduces oestrogen levels. An association between alcohol consumption and breast cancer has been reported in a number of studies; the risk of dying from the disease rises with four or more standard drinks a day, though a causal link has not yet been established.[24]

Women who drink above sensible limits during pregnancy risk miscarrying and tend to deliver smaller babies because alcohol hinders fetal development. The *fetal alcohol syndrome*[25] is rare and confined to women who drink 10 or more standard drinks of alcohol a day; even then, only 4% of infants are affected. It has four components: fetal growth retardation, characteristic facial features, delayed brain development and a variety of congenital abnormalities. The most severely affected children have learning disabilities. Damage occurs during the first few weeks of conception and in the last trimester when brain growth is maximal.

Heavy drinking during pregnancy can result in learning difficulties and behavioural problems in the child: 40% of a group of 14-year-old children who had learning disabilities had been exposed to alcohol.[25] Caution is necessary, however, because such children often come from dysfunctional and socially deprived families, in whom smoking and illicit drug use as well as alcohol is common.

How best to counsel women about drinking during pregnancy? In Britain, the usual advice is to avoid large amounts of alcohol before conception and during the first and third trimesters, otherwise an occasional drink within sensible limits is unlikely to be harmful.[26]

Lungs

Chronic bronchitis, aggravated by heavy smoking, is frequent; there is a fourfold increase in risk of complicating heart failure. *Pneumonia* is five times commoner in heavy drinkers than in the general population, takes longer to resolve and is more often fatal. *Tuberculosis* is a well-recognised scourge of drinkers, especially in those who live rough. Some individuals claim that *bronchial asthma* is aggravated by alcohol; this might be an allergic reaction since alcohol depresses the immune system (see later), or possibly due to bronchoconstriction from acetaldehyde.[27]

Skin, muscle and bones

Bleeding and bruising, either spontaneous due to delayed clotting or associated with accidents, and scarring from falls and accidents when intoxicated, are common in heavy drinkers. The skin of the face tends to be florid with prominent small blood vessels; a red, pustular rash, *acne rosacea*, is seen in some men. People with *psoriasis* find that alcohol in moderate quantities makes the rash worse, and the condition is twice as common in men who drink 12 or more standard drinks a day compared with normal drinkers.[28]

Two types of *myopathy* are related to alcohol.[29] The commoner is a painless chronic muscle weakness with mild wasting, usually affecting the thighs, due to degeneration of muscle fibres and accumulation of triglycerides. It results from years of drinking 12 or more standard drinks a day but improves with abstinence.

Rarely, a dramatic acute form follows a drinking binge. The toxic action of alcohol on muscle cells causes severe pain, generalised cramps and local areas of extremely tender swelling. The products of muscle breakdown are excreted by the kidneys (myoglobinuria) and can lead to renal failure. Recovery over several weeks is usual, though a period of renal dialysis may be required.

Alcohol excess is said to be the commonest cause of *osteoporosis* in men.[30] Thinning of the bones of the spine and pelvis, due to loss of protein and calcium, with backache and sometimes fractures is due to the toxic effect of alcohol on bone cells and alteration in hormones that regulate bone formation. Questions that need answering are whether alcohol contributes to fractured femurs in the elderly and to post-menopausal osteoporosis in women.

Gout, well known in the past as a drinker's complaint, tends to be overlooked today. Recurrent attacks of exquisitely painful arthritis affecting the smaller joints, more common in men than women, are due to deposits of uric acid in the bones. An enquiry should always be made about alcohol use because reduction in intake can have a dramatic effect.

Blood and immune system

Alcohol reduces the number of platelets and increases fibrinolysis, with a resultant tendency to bleeding. It also has a toxic effect on bone marrow and inhibits absorption of folic acid from the gut, both of which delay red cell growth. In some heavy drinkers large, immature red cells, macrocytes, enter the bloodstream so that the *mean corpuscular volume (MCV)* is increased. The normal value is 76–96 fl; figures over 95, in the absence of other causes, should suggest the possibility of heavy drinking, especially if the gamma glutamyl transferase (GGT) is also raised (see p. 33).

The way in which the immune system defends the body against foreign substances is extremely complex. The first line of defence are the T lymphocytes (white blood cells) which recognise and attempt to destroy the foreign invader (cell-mediated immunity); at the same time they activate B lymphocytes to begin producing specific antibodies against the invader (humoral immunity). Recent work suggests that alcohol, beginning at four standard drinks a day, not only suppresses production and therefore numbers of circulating T lymphocytes, but also alters the ability of the immune system to protect the body. This is particularly relevant to virus infections like hepatitis B and C and to human immunodeficiency virus (HIV); the latter, for instance, infects and grows in T lymphocytes. Evidence is not yet available to show that heavy drinkers are more prone to HIV infection or that once infected they are more likely to develop AIDS, but such people, and especially the young, should be warned about a possible risk.[31]

To develop your knowledge in this area, see 'To learn more', p. 250.

Notes

a Thanks and appreciation to Alcohol Concern for permitting reproduction of the body diagram (blank; see p. 25) – student handout G, and body diagram (labelled; see p. 228) – student handout H, from *Teaching About Alcohol Problems: tutor's manual and student handouts*. Compiled by Alcohol Concern, 1987.

b The chemical components of alcohol are commonly recorded thus, $C_2 H_5 OH$. However, this is also referred to as, $CH_3 CH_2 OH$.

Self-assessment questions

1 Many chemicals are alcohols. What is the technical name for the drink we call 'alcohol'?

2. What is the pharmacological action of alcohol?

3. Name three major factors which interact to determine an individual's drinking pattern?

4 At what blood alcohol concentration would you expect a person's judgement to begin to be impaired?

5 What is the name of the enzyme group responsible for breaking down alcohol?

6 Approximately how long would it take to metabolise four pints of beer?

7 How much alcohol would you advise people to drink to reduce the risk of coronary (ischaemic) heart disease?

8 Why do heavy drinkers sometimes develop gout?

9 Name five clinical features accompanying withdrawal from alcohol.

10 Name four conditions for which you would recommend large doses of vitamin B_1 (thiamine), as well as abstinence.

11 What life-threatening condition may accompany drinking in young children and binge drinking?

CHAPTER 5

The young adult

Salme Ahlström

Pre-reading exercise

Spend no more than 15 minutes answering the questions below. When you have read the chapter, repeat the exercise. Do you still feel the same? Has your understanding increased? If so, how?

- Do you think young adults' heavy drinking is most influenced by social norms, socialising, modelling or direct social pressure?
- Does membership of a special sociodemographic group (e.g. social class or religion) have a stronger effect on young adults' drinking patterns than identification with a drinking group?
- Are most of the alcohol-related problems that affect young adults related to chronic heavy drinking or to periodic heavy drinking?
- Would you advise parents and teachers to ban young people from drinking? Or would you encourage them to learn about alcohol-related problems, and to find the best possible ways of preventing them?

Young adults

- Adolescence – the period of transition between childhood and adulthood.
- Social conception of adolescence varies according to the cultural and historical background of the society.
- In most societies, there is a legal minimum age for purchasing alcoholic beverages.

As primarily a social conception, adolescence varies according to the cultural and historical background of the society. Broadly defined, adolescence is the period of transition between childhood and adulthood. It is a time of acquiring the adult skills needed to cope with emotional, economic and social separation from parents and ideally to pave the way for establishing a family, raising children and participating in work and leisure as an independent individual with a separate home and finances.

The interval for which a person occupies young adulthood is obviously problematic to define in terms of exact ages. Despite this, some societies make great efforts to celebrate and ritualise the passage into adolescence and, subsequently, into adulthood. Other societies, meanwhile, are equally well known for their lack of these traditions.

The confirmation, to admit a young person to full membership of the Church, is taken as a social indicator of the onset of adolescence in Protestant societies. The right to vote is commonly taken as a social indicator of the onset of adulthood. Others include the legal right to form new kinship ties by marriage and adoption, to enter the labour force and to drive a motor vehicle, especially a car. In some societies the young adult does not suddenly attain legally competent citizenship with full adult rights all at once on reaching a certain age, but only stepwise over a number of years after the first signs of the onset of adulthood. These signs or indicators often lack consistency and coherence, and are diffuse. In other societies, by contrast, these indicators coincide with a particular point in time and are specific. The conception of young adulthood may be, like its onset, obvious or latent, diffuse or specific, early or late; ambiguity and variability abound, both between and within societies.

In some societies, a legal minimum age for purchasing alcoholic beverages does not exist, though this is exceptional. Some societies set the minimum age limit quite low; in many it is higher for off-premises than on-premises purchases and in some countries the age limit for on-premises consumption is lower when accompanied by parents than when alone or with other young people. In many societies the legal age for purchasing alcohol is lower for beer and wine than for distilled spirits. The United States recently set the highest nationwide age limit in the world: 21 years for all alcoholic beverages.

In most Western industrialised societies young adulthood is taken to span the years 14 to 25. This is the age group referred to by the bulk of the research results, and is thus the focus group of this chapter as well.

Drinking behaviour

Drinking behaviour is affected by:

- social norms
- other social factors
- personality factors
- biological factors
- physical availability of alcoholic beverages
- prices of alcoholic beverages.

Norms determine the incidence and define the limits of socially accepted drinking behaviour. There are right and wrong places to drink, people to drink with, types and amounts of alcoholic beverages to drink, subjects to talk about and activities to pursue while drinking. These various aspects of social influence can also be described as a set of external environmental pressures influencing drinking behaviour, both cognitive and situational.

The past three decades have produced a plethora of reports about sociodemographic influences on young adults' drinking behaviour. However, most research findings have been obtained within a restricted cultural context and narrow time frame and require systematic evaluation. We are also only beginning to understand the impact of the interrelationship between social effects and broader cultural and historical influences on alcohol use.

There is interplay between social norms, other social factors, personality factors and biological factors. In addition, drinking behaviour is affected by the physical availability of alcoholic beverages and by their prices.

Norms, socialising and performance

- Norms determine the incidence and define the limits of socially accepted drinking behaviour.
- Young adults' heavy drinking is influenced:
  - most by social norms of the society
  - secondly by socialising
  - thirdly by modelling
  - only minimally by direct social pressure.
- Young adults want to resemble their peers, therefore:
  - drinking is a performance for others
  - drinkers with companions who consume large amounts of alcohol consume more than others.

Every society has norms for drinking behaviour which carry highly significant implications for determining the incidence and social acceptance of drinking behaviour. These norms vary between different groups, and in any given group they may alter over time and in response to both individual desires and changes in the entire society.

Cognitive social influences include the perception of the other person's behaviour (modelling) and the perceived social norms of other people. *Situational* social influences consist of the direct social pressure in the actual drinking situation and the importance of socialising. The relevance of different types of social influence was evaluated in a Dutch study.[1] Social norms and socialising contributed most to young adults' heavy drinking in public during weekends. Modelling was found the third most influential explanatory variable, but direct social pressure had only minimal influence. Young adults may appreciate the social opportunities drinking situations offer to such an extent that they tend to define drinking itself as a secondary activity to social interaction with other participants.

Dutch young adults did not respond to overt pressures while drinking, but wanted to resemble their peers. For young adults, drinking is not only a matter of personal experimentation, but also a performance for others. Indeed, how the behaviour is likely to be viewed by others may be a more important motivation for behaviour than any personal preference.[2]

In an earlier study, Aitken showed the importance of peers in the drinking behaviour of young adults: drinkers with companions who consumed large amounts of alcohol tended to consume more alcohol and have higher drinking rates than others.[3]

Sociodemographic variation

- Other social factors:
  - gender
  - age
  - social class
  - religion.
- The family formation patterns of young adults have more effect on their drinking patterns than employment, financial circumstances and social position.
- Among employed young adults, 'traditional' women and 'non-traditional' men – in other words those who feel they have substantial obligations at home and intense competition at the workplace – have greater alcohol use than 'non-traditional' women and 'traditional' men.
- Identification with a drinking group has a stronger effect on drinking pattern than membership of a special demographic group.

Social norms, socialising and modelling do not account for all of the observed differences in young adults' behaviour. Other social factors influence their drinking as well: gender, age, social class and religion are all important.

There is considerable evidence that drinking patterns depend somewhat on gender. In every society young men drink more often than young women in the same age category. However, drinking patterns are becoming less differentiated by gender, so that adolescent and young women are now closer to men in their drinking habits than were their mothers and grandmothers. This is a major, ongoing cultural shift in

Western industrialised societies, and in some developing countries. In many societies young adult women consume the largest amount of alcoholic beverages annually. Many of them do not yet have family bonds and responsibilities, which would restrict their leisure-time activities. This period of life is often of great importance for matchmaking, and going to pubs, restaurants, clubs and dance venues is an integral part of it. However, young adult women still drink less, and less frequently, than young adult men, and get drunk less often.

Family responsibilities generally increase when young women get married, and drinking opportunities correspondingly decrease. In societies where drinking wine with meals is a tradition, the annual consumption of alcoholic beverages might be higher among middle-aged than young adult women.

Although young women tend to drink more these days, alcohol consumption remains an expression of masculine identity. The feminine identity, less socially determined than men's, remains incompatible with the image of drunkenness. In moments of success in sports, finance or politics, for example, men are still expected to offer and to drink alcohol.

There is considerable evidence that drinking patterns are also dependent on education, social class, occupation, employment status, region and urbanisation, race/ethnicity and religion, but only a few studies have focused on young adults. Moreover, there are profound differences between societies. For instance, in some countries wine drinking is more popular in rural areas, especially if the country produces wine itself, whereas in Scandinavian countries, for example, drinking occurs mainly in urban settings.

Marriage, parenthood and employment mostly occur in the early part of adulthood and demand the adoption of new social roles. Other transitions generally take place later in life. The role of family formation and dissolution was examined in relation to alcohol consumption in early adulthood in a longitudinal study using data from a large representative British sample.[4] The family formation patterns of young adults were most strongly associated with their current drinking compared with other potential influences such as employment and financial circumstances, social position and well-being. Similarly, in a Dutch study, transitions to parenthood and to marriage at an early age appeared to lead to decreases in alcohol consumption and bouts of heavy drinking.[5] A Norwegian study found that alcohol consumption and use of cannabis were lower among those who had established an adult social role with a partner.[6] This effect was more important than occupation, income and age.

It has been argued that traditional gender roles and gender-role attitudes concerning the division of labour in the family have provided women with a moral or cultural protection against heavier drinking, but that the 'breakdown' of this protection has allowed for greater alcohol use. In a study conducted in the United States, greater alcohol consumption among young women was associated with non-traditional employment and gender-role attitudes concerning responsibilities for household chores and childcare.[7] However, among the employed, the analysis indicated that rather than non-traditional women and traditional men, it is traditional women and non-traditional men who have greater alcohol use – in other words, those who feel they have substantial obligations at home and intense competition at the workplace.

The transition to young adulthood also carries a high risk of unemployment since it involves leaving school and trying to enter working life. The Norwegian researchers found that unemployment was positively related to alcohol consumption and use of cannabis among men, but not women.[6]

The ease of use of sociodemographic variables has overshadowed the importance of the social and collective functions of alcohol consumption. For instance, identification with a drinking group has been shown to be of greater importance than membership of a special demographic group. Drinking groups pressurise even non-permissive people to drink, and light drinkers to drink more heavily than they intended.

Cultural influences

- In wine-producing European countries:
  - the prevalence of drunkenness among young adults is much lower than in Anglo-Saxon and Nordic countries
  - there is a growing trend of separation between eating and drinking
  - drinking to the point of intoxication has become more frequent.

The integration of alcohol with everyday activities can be understood by describing how alcoholic beverages are consumed with meals.[8] In wine-producing countries, drinking is an integral part of a meal. In Italy, drinking between meals is rare; in France it is more common, but in the UK, North America and Nordic countries most drinking takes place outside meals. The importance of meals varies in other dimensions, too. In wine-producing countries, dining is a primary social activity with inherent worth and an integrating function; few people customarily have their evening meal alone. In Anglo-Saxon and Nordic countries, by contrast, eating is conspicuously less of a social ritual; people regard mealtimes as an unavoidable part of their daily routine and spend less time preparing meals and eating.

Young adults' drinking patterns differ in Europe; in wine-producing countries the prevalence of drunkenness is much lower than in Anglo-

Saxon and Nordic countries (see Figure 5.1).[9] Today we are witnessing a growing separation between eating and drinking in France and Italy, especially within the younger generations.[10] Moderate, controlled drinking is being replaced by a more irregular form of drinking tending towards inebriation. Drunken behaviour has become more frequent, less socialised and more anomic than in the festive context. It resembles more the behaviour of young adults in the UK, Denmark and Finland where drinking to the point of intoxication is rather frequent.[11]

Health and social risks

- Most of the alcohol-related problems that affect young adults relate not to chronic heavy drinking, but to periodic heavy drinking and intoxication.

Minorities of young adults, especially males, drink heavily on a regular basis and thereby expose themselves and others to risks. However, most of the alcohol-related problems that affect young adults relate not to

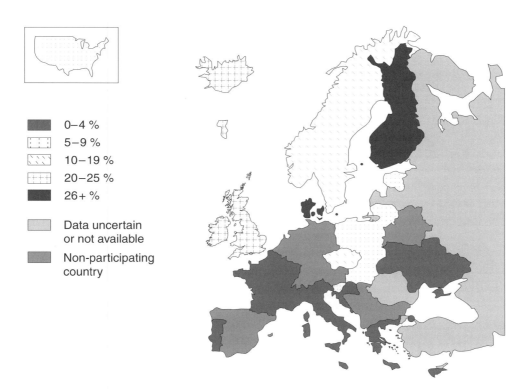

Figure 5.1 Young adults' drinking by country: prevalence of drunkenness. Marked country: limited comparability.

chronic heavy drinking, but to periodic heavy drinking and intoxication. Even the majority of young females who generally drink in moderation may occasionally drink heavily (see Figure 5.2). An illustration of the experienced problems due to alcohol use among Finnish 15–16-year-old students in 1995 is shown in Table 5.1.[12]

Alcohol-related casualties

• Alcohol-related casualties are especially common among younger adults.

Alcohol dulls the faculties, interfering with cognitive, perceptual and motor skills, and more alcohol intensifies these effects. Alcohol is therefore strongly implicated in unintentional injuries and deaths. Partly due to drinking patterns, and partly to less experience and tolerance, alcohol-related casualties are especially common among younger adults in many societies, and a substantial contributor to alcohol-related mortality, particularly when expressed in terms of years of life lost.

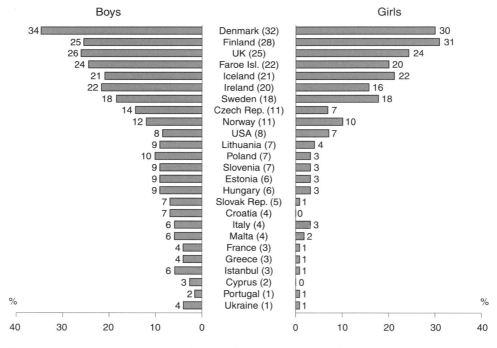

Figure 5.2 Proportion of boy and girls who have been drunk 10 times or more during the last 12 months.

Table 5.1 Experienced problems because of own alcohol use among Finnish students, by gender (% of consumers)[12]

	Boys	Girls
Individual problems		
Reduced performance at school or at work	7	7
Damage to objects or clothing	24	29
Loss of money or other valuable items	16	25
Accident or injury	12	16
Relationship problems		
Quarrel or argument	39	41
Problems in relationship with friends	16	32
Problems in relationship with parents	22	24
Problems in relationship with teachers	3	2
Sexual experiences		
Engaged in unwanted sexual experience	6	10
Engaged in unprotected sex	6	10
Criminal problems		
Scuffle or fight	24	13
Victimised by robbery or theft	1	1
Driving a motorcycle/car under the influence of alcohol	20	4
Trouble with the police	8	7
Subjected to violence	6	4

Drink-driving accidents

• Young drivers have a higher risk due to their inexperience in both driving and drinking.

Alcohol can affect motor skills, balance, visual acuity and reasoning. Drinking therefore tends to increase the risk of harming oneself and others, because of impaired functioning. Such harm can be immediate, as in drink-driving accidents.

Violence

• The relationship between the amount of alcohol consumed and death from violence, both accidental and intentional, is very strong among young adults.

Alcohol is also associated with intentional violence, towards both self and others. Robbery and rape can be predatory crimes in which the intoxicated person becomes the easy victim. More often, the violence arises from drinking in a pub or other context where both the assailant and the victim have been drinking. In many younger populations the net relationship between amount of alcohol consumed and death from violence, both accidental and intentional, is stronger than any other association between drinking and death.

Social problems

- Young adults report more social problems than middle-aged respondents for a given level of drinking.

The variety of alcohol-related social problems includes problems with the family, with friendships and at work, financial difficulties and confrontations with law-enforcement agents. The probability of social consequences rises with the level of drinking.

Risk of illicit drug use, HIV infection and exposure to hepatitis B and C virus

- Heightened risk is associated with:
  - use of intravenous drugs
  - being the partner of an intravenous drug user
  - having homosexual intercourse.
- Use of alcohol and other drugs is related to sexual risk-taking.

The relationship between the use of alcohol, illicit drugs and unprotected sex is complex. Alcohol use can, for some, lead to careless behaviour that could place them at risk of illicit drug use, HIV infection and exposure to hepatitis B and C virus. The epidemiology of HIV and sexually transmitted disease infection indicates that certain behaviours are associated with a heightened risk of becoming infected or infecting one's partner.[13] These include using intravenous drugs, being the partner of an intravenous drug user or of a prostitute, and having homosexual intercourse, especially receptive anogenital intercourse.

Several studies support the view that drinking and non-injected drug use is associated with sexual risk-taking.[14] For instance, an analysis of data from a representative sample of young adults in the US indicates that the use of alcohol and other drugs is related to sexual risk-taking among both men and women after controlling for age, education, family income and other variables.[13] What does emerge from available evidence is that some people take more risks than others, but general theorising is not yet justified in this context. More research is needed to disentangle the mechanisms and processes which may connect different forms of risk-taking among specific subgroups of young adults.[15]

Prevention

Prevention of alcohol-related problems among young people is very challenging. Many young adults expect that drinking alcohol produces positive effects,[9] for example, that they will feel relaxed, happy, more friendly and outgoing, have a lot of fun and be able to forget their problems. However, they are also conscious of the possible negative effects, such as feeling sick, suffering a hangover, harming their health or acting in a regrettable manner.

In countries where the prevalence of drunkenness among young adults is high, the proportion that has positive expectations is higher than in wine-producing countries. In these societies, drunkenness is highly valued among the adult population. Moreover, because young adults like to emulate older adults, they behave according to the cultural norm. Therefore the main aim of prevention should be to change these norms and to make both the adult and young adult population aware of the risks related to drunkenness.

Prevention should be targeted at the environment in which we live. Everybody is a member of some community. Communities provide socialisation of knowledge and values, social control of behaviour, opportunities for social contact and access to social support; they are efficient sites for preventive intervention. Prevention messages can be communicated to individuals and institutions through multiple channels, and behavioural standards can be modelled and enforced through multiple means. Mass media, schools, health institutions, work sites and recreation could all market prevention principles. The impact of multiple, coordinated components of community-based alcohol problem prevention programmes should be synergistic.

To develop your knowledge in this area, see 'To learn more', p. 251.

Self-assessment questions

1 What is the minimum age for purchasing alcoholic beverages in the USA?

2 Young adults' heavy drinking is most influenced by:
   (a) direct social pressure from peers
   (b) social norms of society, or
   (c) modelling?

3 The strongest effect on young adults' drinking patterns is their:
   (a) financial circumstances
   (b) employment
   (c) family formation pattern, or
   (d) social position?

4 Has identification with a drinking group had a strong effect on young adults' drinking patterns?

5 Is the prevalence of drunkenness higher in Anglo-Saxon and Nordic countries than in wine-producing European countries?

6 Has drinking to the point of intoxication become more frequent among young adults in European wine-producing countries?

7 Are most of the alcohol-related problems that affect young adults related to chronic heavy drinking or to periodic heavy drinking and intoxication?

8 Do young drivers have a higher or lower risk for drink-driving accidents than older age groups?

9 Is the relationship between the amount of alcohol consumed and death from violence among young adults weak or strong?

10 Is heightened risk for HIV infection related to the use of intravenous drugs?

CHAPTER 6

Man and woman

Ian MacEwan

Pre-reading exercise

This chapter will explore whether there are differences between men and women in their response to drinking alcohol.

- List what similarities and differences you think there may be for men and women who drink moderately.
- What differences, if any, might you expect between men and women who drink heavily?
- Do you think society has different attitudes towards women who drink? What about women who get into problems with their drinking?
- What differences, if any, might there be between the treatment for men and for women?

Repeat the exercise after reading the chapter to assess if your knowledge is the same, or has improved. This exercise should take no more than 15 minutes to complete.

Gender is not just biological, it is social. Gender issues define the social relations between the sexes, including culturally determined roles for men and women. Thus, social differences between men and women would expect to be reflected in drinking differences between the genders. That these differences are primarily socially determined can be observed in the rapid changes that have occurred in beliefs and behaviours around drinking in the last 50 years. This chapter will therefore explore the different effects of alcohol on men and women.

History

A hundred years ago, heavy drinking of alcohol by men in public places was a dominant mode of the time. Small minorities of women were habitual heavy drinkers, and were regarded as outcasts, criminals and prostitutes: hardly women at all. Most of these women were working class. Although the female crime rate was low compared to the male rate, drunkenness accounted for more than half of women's committals.[1]

While men were allowed considerable behavioural licence, especially in drinking, women were to be mindful of their exemplary roles of wife, mother, guardian of the home and morality. Respectable women did not drink in public, unlike their husbands, although they might have the occasional glass of sherry, claret or home-made fruit wine at home.[2] Along with making or overseeing the food for the household, women also frequently attended to the production of ale, cider and wine – although the consumption of these beverages might not be regarded as drinking.

The community health measures in place then concentrated on men's drunkenness and its consequences of disorder on the streets and disharmony in the home. Early temperance movements drew their membership equally from men and women, only losing most of their male membership as they became supportive of abstinence.[3]

The still commonly held perception of women as secret drinkers is directly linked to the historical relegation of women to the private sphere, and to the notion that respectable women did not drink. Although less overt now than 40 years ago, women, more than men, are still socialised into a set of values concerning responsibility and control. For example, as recently as 1991 a project, *The Place of Alcohol in the Lives of Women*,[4] saw women as responsible, moderate people who nurture, protect, serve and rescue their male partners even from their own folly, and often at the expense of their own needs and preferences. In order to fulfil their responsibilities to their male partners, apparently unencumbered by such notions, women need to be in control of themselves, and this is frequently offered as one of the reasons women do not usually drink heavily. However, this control extends beyond control of self to control of standards in particular social situations and in the wider community. The links between responsibility and control are close and obvious.

These sorts of ideas are current even among young adult girls. Their socially responsible attitudes are more developed than with their male counterparts and are to be applauded. Does it mean that boys leave their drinking responsibility for control in the girls' hands? Many girls answer 'yes'.[5] Drinking culture is a clear example of the problem for women of taking responsibility for others and taking sensible and appropriate action for themselves – a seemingly ageless gender issue.

In all cultures whose drinking practices have been recorded, men are more likely than women to drink, drink larger quantities, drink more frequently and report more drinking-related problems.[6]

The gender differences in drinking and heavy drinking rates are paralleled by gender differences in the prevalence of clinical assessments of drink-related problems. While more men than women are assessed with these problems, the ratios vary considerably between cultures. The lower rates for women do not mean that women's drinking is inconsequential.

Understanding more about the differences between men's and women's drinking can increase knowledge about the factors that influence drinking behaviour and drinking problems. Trying to understand why women as a group drink less than men can help to clarify how gender and gender roles (for example, social expectations about how women and men should behave) affect the drinking behaviour of both women and men.

Men and women: similarities

There are marked similarities between men's and women's drinking patterns. The younger of both genders have higher rates of consumption and problems than the older adult. The younger tend to engage more in binge or episodic drinking styles and to suffer the consequences of alcohol-related car crashes.[7]

For both genders, those who are divorced or separated, never-married or lesbian or gay male show higher rates of drinking and related problems.[8] Studies show that drinking can be the cause, consequence or accompaniment for any of these states, except for sexual orientation, which may influence alcohol consumption but not the reverse. Interestingly, dissolution of partnership has led to a decrease in problem drinking for women, perhaps by removing the woman from a relationship in which partnership problems and excessive drinking were mutually reinforcing.[9]

A study examining the relationship between heavy drinking and violence offences found no significant differences between men and women.[10]

The genetic component in predisposition to alcohol dependence is probably as strong in men as in women.[11]

Men and women: differences in drinking

In a major randomised study of over 4000 drinking adults:[12]

- 73% of the alcohol was consumed by men
- the median annual consumption reported by male drinkers was 7.4 litres of absolute alcohol – this is equivalent to 500 cans of beer a year, or a little over nine cans a week
- the 2.1 litre median reported by women drinkers is equivalent to about 140 glasses of beer or 140 ml glasses of wine a year, or a little under three cans of beer or glasses of wine a week
- the top 10% of drinkers were predominantly male
- for men drinkers the median frequency of drinking was about once every two to three days, while for women drinkers it was once every five or six days

- 19% of male drinkers and 10% of female drinkers were drinking every day
- on a typical drinking occasion, men consumed the equivalent of three cans of beer and women two glasses of wine
- when asked how often they consumed six or more drinks, almost three-quarters of male drinkers stated that they did so at least once a year, 41% monthly and 21% weekly
- when women drinkers were asked how often they consumed four or more drinks, 57% said they did so at least annually, 22% at least monthly and 8% at least weekly
- 31% of male drinkers and 14% of female drinkers drank enough to feel drunk at least once a month, while for 13% of men and 4% of women this occurred at least weekly
- men accounted for over two-thirds of reports of drunkenness.

In the United Kingdom, the 1997 Omnibus Survey[13] found that:

- on average, men drank 15.9 standard drinks of alcohol a week – almost eight pints of beer or the equivalent in other types of drink. Women's consumption was much lower at 6.9 standard drinks on average
- 70% of men and 58% of women had drunk alcohol in the previous seven days. About one in five men and one in 10 women had had a drink on five or more days
- one in five men had drunk more than eight standard drinks on at least one day in the previous week. The proportion that had done so varied sharply with age, ranging from 5% of men aged 65 and over, to as many as 39% of young men aged 16–24.
- women were much less likely than men to drink heavily – 8% had drunk more than six standard drinks on at least one day in the previous week
- 8% of men and 3% of women said they got at least slightly drunk every week
- 16% of men drinkers and 11% of women drinkers said that at some time they had tried to cut down their drinking for health reasons.

A number of studies[14] indicate that sons tend to adopt the drinking pattern of their father and daughters of their mother.

A Canadian study[15] suggests that many gender differences in drinking patterns are dependent on age and marital status. As men and women get older, and especially after settling into a stable relationship, men change their drinking behaviour towards the behaviour of their female partner.

A representative sample of adults revealed that 24% of male lifetime drinkers and 15% of female lifetime drinkers met the DSM-IV criteria for sometime alcohol dependence.[16]

Gender differences were analysed in a sample of 233 problem drinkers treated at the same clinic.[17] Demographic and family history measures showed a few gender differences. Men reported more alcohol consumption than did women, but patterns of drinking and intoxication levels were similar.

Males reported drinking and intoxication at an earlier age, more beer and less wine drinking, and more drinking away from home and driving after drinking. Women reported more negative emotional effects of drinking and more spouses with alcohol problems. Despite similar problem duration, men showed more lifetime alcohol problems but not dependence signs. Men were more likely to accept a disease concept of alcoholism.[18] Rates of smoking, other drug use and other life problems were similar.

Women: gender-specific issues

Until the last two decades alcohol and drug problems were less evident among women than men. Most research and literature described the male stereotype. As greater numbers of women have taken on new roles in paid employment and begun to access positions of public power and influence, more attention has been directed to issues that are specific to women.

Drinking is now more socially acceptable for women and alcohol is more commonly used as a means of managing stress and coping with personal and social pressures than the prescription drugs that have previously been preferred.

In the 1960s the female:male ratio for problems with alcohol was 1:10; now it is 1:2.5.[19] Similarly, the ratio presenting to treatment services is diminishing as the prevalence of problems increases, stigma decreases and services become more accessible. Alcohol-related problems seem to be increasing, particularly for young women.

Women are physiologically more vulnerable to alcohol because of the lower volume of distribution of the substance in the female with a higher percentage of body fat.[20] Diminished levels of gastric alcohol dehydrogenase in women may also play a part.[21] Vulnerability to liver disease is important.[22] Any alcohol use is now thought to be a risk factor for breast cancer in women.[23] Women need to be particularly careful during pregnancy. Alcohol crosses the placenta and can be damaging to the fetus. Fetal alcohol syndrome is a cluster of birth defects caused by heavy drinking during pregnancy. Even a single occasion may put the fetus at risk.[24]

The influence of a partner's drinking is much greater for women than it is for men. This may be an imitation of the drinking behaviour of a dominant male. Not just conformity but also discrepancies in the drinking patterns of male–female partners may increase a person's risk for problem drinking. This is also evidenced in same-sex relationships. Partners (of either sex) report more intoxication and adverse drinking consequences if they perceive discrepancies between their own and their partner's drinking than if they perceived their drinking pattern as similar.[9] It is unclear whether discrepant drinking patterns of partners reflect conflicts in a relationship, cause them, or both.

Women develop alcohol-related problems more quickly than men. There is conflicting research evidence[25] as to why this is. Some suggest alcohol problems for women become more acute faster than for men and that the deterioration in functioning is exposed more clearly because the stigma has decreased and the access to services increased. Others suggest that women are more open than men to admitting having problems and are therefore more identifiable.

Although women may be experiencing alcohol/drug-related problems, their understanding of these is more likely to be in terms of their experience of depression, loss, grief, anxiety, fear or frustration. Alcohol/ drug use is seen, more clearly for women than for men, as a way of coping with these experiences.

Statistically,[26] we know that women in relation to men are more likely to:

- misuse medication in addition to alcohol/drugs
- start drinking alcohol regularly later in life
- have a shorter prehistory of alcohol/drug dependence
- drink alone more often
- have a partner who also has an alcohol/drug dependence
- have sole responsibility for care of children
- report guilt feelings about their drinking more often
- have lower self-esteem
- experience greater feelings of helplessness about their problems
- more often report anxiety and depression
- attempt suicide more often.

Femininity does not endorse binge drinking as a rite of passage to adulthood as being loud, unruly or sick is not feminine;[27] unlike smoking, which is an anticipatory rite of passage for young females as it does not undermine one's femininity as control and sophistication can be maintained.[28]

Men: gender-specific issues

Studies [27,29] have shown that in some social groups young males have low self-esteem to such a level that they are apprehensive about contact with women even when they are attracted to them. For these males, aged 17 to 27, it is much less threatening for them to remain within the confines of the male peer group where they are accepted than to venture into the world of women. Priority is with the male peer group. Women, even wives and girlfriends, are seen as a threat to the group as they compete for members' time and attention. Alcohol is used as a tool to boost their confidence and to help them combat their apprehension in dealing with women. Hostility and negativity towards women are reflected in the ways in which women are referred to in a sexist and aggressive manner.

Archer, in her study,[30] found that young males who frequently got drunk did not have steady girlfriends and were less influenced by females. She also found that the males in her study appeared to be unaware of the type of responsible drinking behaviour that females admired.

Drinking is both the major focus of these male-only groups and a symbol of their inclusion. In order to feel part of the group the male has to fit in with the group's drinking pattern.

There does not appear to be the same peer pressure on females to consume alcohol as there is with males.[27] Young women's consumption correlates comparatively strongly with self-efficacy in different moods and social norms. However, females tend to drink at a faster rate when in mixed-sex groups rather than in groups of females only.[31] This may reflect the influence of the males on drinking behaviour, especially if they are older than the females.

For young males, getting drunk is a rite of passage to adulthood and an immense bonding experience – a few beers with the boys.[27] Males and females who have predominantly androgenous traits seem to have lower alcohol consumption and higher self-esteem. It appears that it is when males and females try to live up to stereotypical feminine or masculine images that the problems occur.[27]

Gender differences in response to treatment

Gender differences relating to alcohol treatment are receiving increased attention.[32] Studies of women in treatment[33] show that in comparison with men they will more often ask for help in identifying their own anger and in expressing aggression in adequate ways, in learning to distinguish between their own and others' feelings, and in ensuring satisfaction of their own needs in a responsible way. This includes training in asking for things directly and in learning to stand up for one's own rights in conflict situations.

Women, more often than men, will ask that treatment addresses issues such as marital problems, parental roles, child-care questions, sexuality and self-assertion. Women will also request that treatment be more human-oriented and less problem-substance focused.[34]

Too often controlled drinking programmes (which aim for reduction in drinking rather than abstinence) are focused on what are perceived as male goals, for example reduction in consumption. Female goals might reflect other foci such as reducing drinking alone; follow-on support; addressing non-substance issues, particularly a heavy drinking/drug-using partner; financial and family pressures; low self-esteem; or trauma related to sexual abuse.[35]

Women tend to respond better to self-help programmes or to treatment in women-only groups. After receiving traditional treatments, women do better in the short term but men do better after one year. This reflects the male orientation of most traditional treatment programmes which tend to use psychotherapy, milieu therapy and 12-step programmes. Women do better with their treatment goals when there is a greater emphasis on a cognitive-behavioural orientation, which is less common.

Women appear to do better in controlled drinking programmes than men. Men tend to have better outcomes in peer-oriented groups, perhaps because men's camaraderie in drinking may find its substitutions in group therapy within treatment or self-help groups such as Alcoholics Anonymous (AA).[18]

Women respond better in same-gender rather than in mixed-gender groups. In all-female groups, women tend to talk more and to be more self-revealing; in mixed-gender groups they tend to interact less both with the men and with other women, while the men seem to benefit in that they talk about their feelings more when women are present.[36]

Women may have poorer outcomes at long-term follow-ups because up to one third of them live with a heavily drinking spouse. Studies[37] indicate only between 10% and 15% of male problem drinkers live with a heavy drinking spouse. Women report significantly less support for entering treatment from their partners than do males. Women's family responsibilities and pressure from partners may cause them to drop out of treatment or give up on their treatment goals more quickly than males.

When men and women, after treatment, give up on an abstinence goal, women drink less, and less often, than men.[38] However, women drink to intoxication more than men. Men relapse alone more often than women. Men and women report relapsing frequently with same-sex friends and women show a tendency to relapse in the presence of romantic partners. Men also tend to report more positive mood states during relapse than women, which is congruent with the finding that women report more depression.

Other factors

The major consequences of excessive alcohol use for an individual may be biological (physical dependence, neuropsychological defects, physical illnesses such as pancreatitis and cirrhosis), psychological (depression, anxiety, cognitive dysfunction) or social (relationship dysfunctions, job difficulties, legal problems). Two of the major consequences that are gender specific are employment factors for women and sexual problems for men and women.

Employment

Prior to the 1970s employment outside the home was considered to affect women's mental health and drinking behaviour adversely, especially when combined with marital or family roles. Findings since then have indicated otherwise. Although women working outside the home consume more than those inside the home, there is not a higher incidence of heavy drinking or alcohol-related problems.

On the contrary, lack of and loss of outside work has been associated with higher rates of problem drinking. However, an exception occurs for women drinkers employed in occupations with more than 50% male workers – they score higher on a problem-drinking index than women drinkers in a workforce with more female workers.[39]

The influence of gender composition of co-workers on drinking behaviour seems to be specific for women. Men's drinking behaviour does not seem to be affected by this factor. Interpretations of the heavier drinking of those women in male-oriented occupations include the imitation of the male drinking style, more drinking opportunities, stress related to a minority status in male-dominated occupations, and the use of drinking as a symbolic expression of power and gender equality.[40]

Unemployment, relationship difficulties and childless but wanting children are likely to lead to increased drinking in women but not in men. The reason for this gender difference is not fully understood.

Sexual problems

Both women and men expect alcohol to enhance sexual experience. Sexual problems are the strongest single predictors of continued problem drinking for both men and women,[41] for example impotency in men and lack of libido in women.

Conclusion

While there are a few similarities in the alcohol use of men and women, there are substantial differences. Treatment should reflect these differences and take account of the special needs of each gender.

For women:

- treatment needs to focus on understanding the factors behind problem drinking, rather than on male-oriented goals such as reduction of consumption
- women-only treatment groups need to be made available as these enable women to both express themselves more freely and sustain a longer-term recovery
- extra support needs to be provided for women in treatment as they are much less likely than their male counterparts to be receiving outside support from their partners.

For men:

- a primary focus on reduction of consumption is helpful
- the provision of male-only groups which may simulate the camaraderie of a drinking group has worked effectively in treatment.

For both young men and women there is an urgent priority: the continued provision of responsible drinking messages directed at young adults to counteract the higher rates of consumption and problems experienced by this group in comparison to previous generations.

To develop your knowledge in this area, see 'To learn more', p. 254.

Self-assessment questions

1 Has the drinking of men and of women changed over the last 100 years?
2 Have community health measures with regard to men and to women's drinking changed over the last 100 years?
3 Are there differences in attitudes towards drinking between young adult males and females?
4 Are there differences between cultures in who drinks more: men or women?
5 Which experiences common to men and women have shown higher rates of drinking and related problems?
6 Are men more physiologically vulnerable to alcohol than women?
7 Generally speaking, are men or are women more likely to be socially influenced in their drinking pattern?

8 Is it true that less importance is given to gender differences in drinking these days?
9 Do men or do women respond better to self-help groups?
10 Are women employed outside the home drinking more than women inside the home?

CHAPTER 7

The importance of the family

Richard Velleman

Pre-reading exercise

Two **case studies** are briefly described below. Start this chapter by reading the case studies and then, before reading on, think about these individuals and their stories that are so briefly encapsulated.

Now do the following two exercises. Spend no more than 10 minutes on each.

1 List the main issues **for the family member** that you can see in these case studies.
2 List the main issues **for helpers** – professionals or others – who are trying to help family members deal with someone else in the family with an alcohol problem.

The questions that we collectively need to address are:

1 How can we understand a family's experience?
2 What should we do to help family members?

Of course, not everyone describes such a violent interaction with a problem-drinking relative; but it is also a fact that both of these awful (and true) stories are very typical of what family members often endure.

You were previously asked to address the questions of 'How can we understand a family's experience, and what should we do to help family members?' This chapter will put forward a framework that will allow us to answer these questions.

CASE STUDY: FRANK

Frank is eight years old, with two younger sisters. Frank is often left to look after his younger siblings while his father is out, at the pub. His father is a very heavy drinker; and his mother left the family two years ago due to the heavy drinking and violence that she received. Frank's father mainly takes the violence out on Frank now. Frank's father, however, conceals this violent side to his behaviour, being an immensely charming man outside the family.

Frank gets withdrawn and distracted at school, and is often naughty and disruptive. He often comes to the attention of the head teacher because of this. One day Frank tells his teacher about the violence he receives at home. His teacher is aghast, and worried, and tells the head. The head decides to confront Frank's father.

Frank's father ('Mr Charm himself' says the now adult Frank) charms the head ('You know what a naughty boy Frank is – he is always being disruptive and telling fibs'), and the head is embarrassed at being 'taken in' by Frank. Frank's father insists that the head punish Frank for 'telling lies', and then later punishes Frank himself, far more brutally, for betraying him. Frank never tells anyone again, until he talks to me as an adult.

CASE STUDY: SYLVIA[a]

Sylvia is in her mid-fifties, and had been married to a problem-drinking husband. When the children were very young, he started being violent towards Sylvia: 'very violent – he hit me lots of times'. She 'had to wear a cardigan or a jumper all the time [to hide] where he'd poked and prodded me'. Sylvia recalled one night 'it was absolutely terrible, he started smashing everything in the bedroom and throwing it out. I was so frightened I went and stood in the children's bedroom; it went on for hours and hours, and then he started in the sitting room. I didn't know what to do – whether to get the children out [they were asleep] or to leave them'.

Sylvia described herself as 'living in fear 24 hours a day' as her husband became increasingly violent. He would come into the kitchen 'and make me stand to attention and look into his eyes. If I said anything out of place or defiant at all he'd hit me; I was frightened'. She went to her GP who put her on tranquillisers ('I know his attitude was, "silly woman, what's she doing here?"').

Eventually she divorced her husband after 16 years of marriage.

The context

Drinking alcohol is often an enjoyable experience. Alcohol is used within many cultures in a huge variety of ways – to signify a celebration, to make a toast, to give a lift to a party, to commiserate with someone, to reduce social anxiety and so on. We all recognise that alcohol can be the mainstay of family celebrations and social life – the relaxing drink after work, the convivial glass with friends over dinner or down at the pub, the toast at a wedding or major celebration. 'What would you like to drink?' is often the first question at social gatherings, whether within or outside the home.

Most people in Britain drink alcohol at some time or another in any year. A good proportion of them drink alcohol on a weekly basis, or more frequently. Part of the reason that alcohol is so widely used is that it is a psychoactive drug. The reason that it does lift a party or reduce social anxiety is that it has strong effects on the brain: for example, alcohol tends to reduce social inhibitions. Unfortunately, the very fact that alcohol is a psychoactive drug means that it is also associated with a wide range of problems.

It is of course true that many people who drink alcohol, even on a regular basis, experience no problems in relation to this use. Nevertheless, some people do have problems. Some people become dependent on the inhibition-reducing elements, and start relying on alcohol as opposed to acquiring the skills to overcome anxiety without the use of alcohol. Other people start to drink habitually, and then discover that the effects of stopping drinking are uncomfortable or painful. Alcohol is an addictive substance, and withdrawing off it is problematic. For others, their drinking leads them to physical ill health, problems with their livers, with their stomachs and so on (see Chapter 4); and for others, drinking is associated with antisocial behaviour, such as fighting or criminal activity. In fact, alcohol is associated with a myriad of problems: at work, with friends, with the law, with aggression and violence.[1] In addition, with many people, their drinking affects their families even more than it affects the drinkers.

Over the years helping services have been developed to try to aid people who have problems with their own drinking. There exists, across the UK, networks of help which include NHS in-patient and community teams, specialist social workers, non-statutory agencies (often known as alcohol advisory centres) in most counties and in many smaller administrative units, and self-help groups such as Alcoholics Anonymous.

For some reason, *families* who are affected by the drinking of one of their members are generally ignored by service providers. This is all the more strange given the fact that:

• family members often suffer many negative experiences, including violence, poverty and social isolation

- family members will often develop problems because of these experiences
- some will be individual problems (such as anxiety and depression)
- others will be family problems (such as breakdowns in such family structures and systems as rituals, roles, routines, communication structures, social life and finances)
- children may have particular difficulties, demonstrating whilst still young a higher propensity for antisocial behaviour, emotional problems and problems in the school environment; and during adolescence, often showing friendship difficulties, a division between home life and peer relationships, being prescribed psychoactive drugs, earlier use of alcohol or drugs, leaving home early, earlier marriages and involvement with a 'semi-deviant' subculture.

The strange thing is that, although many family members of people with alcohol problems do have such extremely high physical and psychological morbidity (see, for example, references 2 or 3), they generally seem to be invisible, both to primary healthcare professionals and to specialist substance misuse agencies alike.

Why do family members develop these problems?

Some of the main reasons why family members develop problems in response to someone else's drinking behaviour is that the drinking itself will often impact on the family as a whole, in terms of affecting family structures. Common areas are shown in Box 7.1.

However, the reasons why family members develop problems in response to someone else's drinking behaviour are not just about changes in family structure. The problem drinker, and other people in the household, also change their behaviour. The problem drinker may become more violent (either towards their partner, or towards their children), and even if they do not show physical violence they may well become more aggressive or argumentative. Or they may become more withdrawn from the family. Alternatively, they may demonstrate an unpredictable combination of these – violent sometimes, withdrawn at others, over-affectionate at other times and just 'normal' the rest of the time. And others in the family, who do not have problems with their own drinking, may also be affected. Many children are at a loss to understand why their non-problem-drinking parent's behaviour becomes so 'odd', not understanding that they may be becoming increasingly preoccupied with their problem-drinking partner, or increasingly hostile towards them; or that, in the

Box 7.1 Problems in family structure

Family rituals

These are things which define the occasion or the day as being special, and different from other days and occasions. Often these occasions are especially important precisely in the sense of being designed or expected to cement family relationships. Obvious examples are Christmas celebrations, birthdays, weddings and so forth.

Family roles

Alcohol misuse tends to change the roles played by family members in relation to one another, and to the outside world. Most families operate some form of division of labour – one person managing the family's finances, the other supervising the children, one doing the gardening, the other doing the cooking, and so on. But as one member of the family develops more of a drink problem, the other members are likely to find themselves having to take over his or her role themselves. Eventually, one member may be performing all the roles – finances, disciplining, shopping, cleaning, household management, and so on.

Family routines

Another likely consequence of problem drinking is that the drinker's behaviour becomes unpredictable, and naturally this makes it very difficult for the family as a whole to plan anything in advance or to stick to familiar routines. Will he or she be in a fit state to collect the child from school? What time will he or she come home, and in what state? Should meals be served up or not? Clearly, this sort of constant uncertainty can be highly disruptive, and it helps to explain a commonly found paradox in the families of problem drinkers: that while the problem drinker may be withdrawing from the family – by no longer playing the role within it that he or she did previously – he or she nonetheless appears to dominate it.

Family communication

A fourth area of family functioning which is often affected by alcohol and alcohol misuse relates to the kind of communication that takes place between family members. It may be that the partner with the problem refuses to talk about it, even though it is clearly beginning to dominate his or her, and the family's, life. Alternatively, alcohol may loosen the tongue and things might be said which would not have been said in a sober state. Or again, alcohol can itself perhaps become the main topic of conversation – has he or she been drinking again, if so how much and with what effect, who is going to telephone the boss to say that s/he won't be in because s/he's got flu yet again, and so forth.

Family social life

Most people who have a parent or partner with a drinking problem find talking about it to others to be extraordinarily difficult. The problem is often simply seen as being too shameful to admit. Yet a result of the difficulty of explaining the situation to other people is that the family tends to withdraw into itself. The high degree of social embarrassment involved, and the unpredictability so often associated with drinking problems, makes it very awkward to extend invitations to others to visit the family home, or to accept invitations to visit theirs or to attend other social gatherings. The family thus tends to become increasingly socially isolated.

Family finances

Financial problems are a further major strain for the family. Most obviously, money which is spent on drink is not available for other kinds of family expenditure; but it may also be that a drink problem results in the family's income being greatly diminished (for example, if the drinker loses his or her job). There follow all sorts of knock-on consequences: the rent or the mortgage repayments may not be paid, debts may be run up, accommodation may be lost, power may be cut off. Clearly, such problems in themselves can have dire consequences for children in such families.

absence of their partner as someone who takes a share of the household tasks, the one sober parent has to take on the role of being the only disciplinarian, or the only bringer of bad news.

How to make a bad situation worse!

Looking at these situations from the child's point of view, the evidence is that, although living in a home with a parent with a drinking problem is often a big difficulty, some things in the family can make things even worse. Box 7.2 lists some of the issues that can make a bad situation worse.

Box 7.2 How to make a bad situation for a child even worse

- Violence – even if it is not directed at the child
- Marital conflict – the major concern of the child
- Separation, divorce and parent loss
- Inconsistency and ambivalence in parenting
- All of these elements lead to unpredictability, which leads to many difficulties:
    - a deteriorating parent – child relationship
    - diminishing feelings of self-esteem
    - social isolation
    - feelings of exclusion

Research into the upbringing of children in general suggests that unpredictability is the single most important factor impairing children's ability to lead successful and healthy childhoods and adulthoods, and it is a large part of the explanation of why children brought up in care fare worse than other children.[4] In problem-drinking families, unpredictability leads to many difficulties – a deteriorating parent–child relationship, diminishing feelings of self-esteem, and social isolation and feelings of exclusion.

One of the most fundamental human needs is to be able to impose some sort of order on what is happening, to be able to understand and explain. This allows people, to some extent, to predict what is going on in order to be able to come to terms with it. The children of problem drinkers know that things are going wrong, that in some way they are 'different'. A simple and obvious explanation is that they are to blame, that they are in some way responsible for their parents' drinking and drug-taking and for what happens in consequence of it. It is easy to see why self-blame and low self-esteem are very common in children of problem-drinking and drug-using parents.

From recent research looking at children who grow up in these circumstances[5] it seemed that, given the often very difficult circumstances of their early years, two common patterns for adolescents emerged. One of them had adolescents being relatively socially isolated, perhaps being prescribed psychoactive medication for 'anxiety' or 'depression', trying to escape from their family home, leaving home earlier, getting into long-term relationships earlier and getting married earlier. The other involved adolescents having strong peer relationships but keeping them very isolated from their family of origin, becoming involved in drinking and drug-taking at a young age, becoming involved with a semi-deviant subculture and possibly becoming more involved with antisocial activity.

Clearly, these are huge generalisations and many children acted in neither (or indeed both) of these ways.

Children, then, can be very badly affected by a parental drinking problem. Yet this is not a necessary consequence. There are things that clearly make the problems worse for children (and indeed for other family members). But there are also things that can make the situation far better for relatives, and which reduce the risk of a negative outcome for the child.

Resilient people: what protects relatives from harm?

The range of detrimental effects outlined above are not *certain* to occur. There are factors that make them *less* likely to occur, even if one parent or partner has a drinking problem. These are shown in Box 7.3.

There are a range of 'protective factors' which tend to make children more resilient and more able to cope with problems in their family of origin or in their family lives when they grow to adulthood. Some of these factors are associated with how the family of origin functions with someone with a drinking problem in its midst. These factors include *the other parent*: how the non-problem-drinking parent reacts is crucial. If he or she is able to provide a stable environment where the child can grow and develop, and is able to provide the time and attention which so many children require, the risks of a negative outcome are reduced.

Similarly, the second factor is a *cohesive parental relationship*: the important issue to children is the quality of the family environment, as opposed to the parental problem drinking. If parents manage to retain their cohesive relationship and present a united and caring front to the children, the children will be less at risk.

Third, a *cohesive family*: even if the parents do not manage to retain the cohesion within their own relationship, risk will be reduced if family *relationships*, family *affection* and family *activities* are maintained.

Fourth, if the children are able to separate family life from the disruptive behaviour of the problem drinker (for example, if they are able to preserve distinct family rituals [see Box 7.1]), they are more likely to grow to adulthood with fewer problems.

Many of these 'protective' factors lie within the family of origin, but some are external support systems which lie outside of it. One such factor is the influence of important others, outside of the family, usually a *non-parental adult*. The stabilising influence mentioned earlier does not have to come from the other parent: another figure can provide it, such as a grandparent, an influential teacher or a neighbour.

Box 7.3 Resilience: what protects relatives from harm?

As children

Within the family of origin: Outside the family of origin:

- the other parent

- cohesive parental relationship

- cohesive family

- separation of family life from the disruptive behaviour of the problem drinker

- other important influences, e.g. a non-parental adult
- disengagement from the disruptive elements of family life
- engagement with others outside the family
- 'planning' or 'deliberateness'

As adults
- 'planning' or 'deliberateness'
- selection of a partner and forming a new family
- deliberate attempt to select positive family rituals

Another protective factor relates to how actively the child both *disengages* from the disruptive elements of family life and *engages* with others outside the family (e.g. schoolmates) or with stabilising activities (such as a major hobby). A third relates to a notion termed by some writers as *'planning'* or *'deliberateness'* – the active and deliberate attempt to make one's life more ordered and structured, and less disrupted by the problems in the family.

These factors can all lead to resilience, in that they can produce *attachment* and *security* as opposed to unpredictability, insecurity, exclusion and isolation.

The ability to protect oneself from problems within one's family of origin can continue into adulthood as well. Factors which have been found to enable adults from highly disrupted environments to cope adequately with adult life include – *'planning'* or *'deliberateness'* again, the *selection of a stable partner*, the *forming a new family* and the *deliberate attempt to select positive family rituals* to work out with one's partner which components of the rituals of both families of origin the new family wishes to retain, and which they wish to dispense with.

So how can we help family members?

The children and other family members of problem drinkers will often have serious problems of their own. In children, these problems will be especially apparent while they are still children and sometimes will continue into adulthood. Children and other family members often need help to enable them to deal with such problems. Yet, almost all specialised services only help the problem drinkers, not their families. This is not to question that those with problems with their own drinking need help. Nevertheless, the lack of services for the children and other family members of problem drinkers show that, largely, they are the forgotten and ignored victims of the misuse of alcohol.

There are many ideas for helping family members; this chapter will just focus on a few. Further ideas are contained in references 5, 6 and 7.

Designated services for children

It seem self-evident that there is a need for more designated services aimed at family members in general, and the children of problem drinkers in particular. These services are rare, and of those that do exist, almost all of the ones that serve children have policies which necessitate *informing parents* about the fact that the children have asked for help. Clearly, if the reason that the child wants help is to talk about how best to cope with a sometimes violent parent, the *last thing* that child may want is for the parent to be informed that the child has asked for help!

So, services which could escape the need to inform parents of the child's attendance are needed. These services could do a great deal:

- they could offer a listening ear, enabling the child to feel that at least *someone* was prepared to listen, and to hear
- they could also provide counselling, enabling the child to work through the various options open to him or her as to how best to cope with a problem-drinking parent, and to assess which option might be the best one to pursue for that particular child in that particular situation.

Alcohol services: specialised team member for work with children

As a minimum, agencies that deal with alcohol problems should, as a matter of course, widen their net and make their counselling services available to children and other family members affected by a parent's alcohol use. They should also designate one or more members of their team to specialise in work with children and to set up cross-referral systems, and joint working, with school counselling and child psychology and psychiatry services.

Generic services for children: awareness of parental problem drinking

Similarly, generic services for children and families need to be aware that parental alcohol problems are extremely prevalent, and hence many difficulties presented by children may have this parental problem as an underlying causative factor. Often such parents will be very resistant to revealing their problems, of course, and an important training need for staff within children's services may be the issue of how to raise these topics in an unthreatening manner.

Biggest single issue: confidentiality

The biggest issue for services for children and families, however, is that of confidentiality: how to allow children to express their problems to professionals without these professionals either immediately involving the parents of the child, or invoking child protection procedures.

Will these ideas involve everyone learning many new skills?

The simple answer is 'no'! Working with children and other family members requires the same set of skills as people already have in their work with problem drinkers, or with any other client group, as shown in Box 7.4.

Conclusion

People with drinking problems often claim that it does not affect their families. This is not true. Living with a problem drinker can affect other family members, particularly children, in many quite negative ways.

Three additional points can be made. First, *any* person's behaviour with respect to alcohol affects and influences the family. Children learn most of their attitudes and behaviours concerning alcohol from their parents; and partners in relationships are also influenced by someone's drinking habits.

Box 7.4 The basic skills of helping

Helpers need to be:

- warm, empathic and genuine

and to be able to:

- make a therapeutic relationship
- help clients explore their difficulties
- enable clients to set achievable goals
- empower clients to take action to reach these achievable goals
- stay with clients and help them stabilise and maintain changed behaviours, thoughts and emotions

---

Second, this influence is not always negative. Sometimes it can be very positive, as when partners influence each other in moderate as opposed to excessive patterns, and children learn about sensible drinking and are not given an example of inappropriate use. But behaviour in relation to drinking *always* will influence, and therefore affect, the attitudes and behaviour of other family members.

Third, when this influence is negative it is very powerful indeed, able dramatically and adversely to affect the lives of all family members, sometimes over quite long periods of their lives. An important priority must be to develop services which adequately help these family members.

To develop your knowledge in this area, see 'To learn more', p. 254.

Self-assessment questions

1 What are some of the main difficulties that alcohol problems can cause for family members?
2 What types of problem often arise in family structures?
3 What are the key issues that make a bad situation worse?
4 What are the key protective issues which often lead to resilience?
5 Why is stability so important?
6 What are the main ways family members can be helped?
7 What are the key skills needed to help family members?

Note

a This case study comes from the book: Velleman R, Copello A and Maslin J (eds) (1998) *Living With Drink: women who live with problem drinkers*. Longmans, London.

CHAPTER 8

The older adult

Eileen McKee

In this chapter, you will learn about:

- the meaning of alcohol to an older person
- problematic consumption patterns:
    - typology   – chronic
                       – reactive
- identification:
    - comparison between younger and older problematic consumers
    - activities of daily living (ADL)
    - tools to assist with identification
    - who identifies
    - behavioural, verbal and visual indicators

- treatment:
    - roles of worker
    - termination guidelines
    - evaluation

- concurrent issues to investigate:
    - elder abuse
    - gambling
    - home detoxification
    - consultation to professional and non-professional caregivers.

This chapter will offer an introduction to alcohol use and older adults. The material is designed to address the needs of health, spiritual and social care professionals who wish to develop a basic understanding of alcohol and the older person. Treatment approaches and interventions appropriate to this population will be presented.

The meaning of alcohol to an older person

It is difficult to say, in general terms, what alcohol means to any one person. However, there are general distinctions in the meaning of alcohol to specific cultures and subcultures.[1] For some, it is a rite of passage, or the symbol of adulthood or manhood. For others, alcohol consumption can be an attribute or a deficit. The value may vary with the age and gender of the consumer, with the type of alcohol, and with the circumstances under, and era in, which it is consumed. The meanings can vary, symbolising celebration, health, virility, status, romance or relaxation. For example, to underage high-school students, drinking beer together can mean sexual prowess, manhood, acceptance by peers, avoidance of ridicule or defiance of authority. In contrast, to mature factory workers at the end of the shift, drinking beer together can mean relaxation, a reward, camaraderie and refreshment. Alcohol can also mean devastation, pain and moral weakness. In summary, the meaning of alcohol is the product of the specific personal and social context of each episode.

For an ageing person, the meanings may be entrenched over many years, even decades, of consumption. Age can also increase the need for a stable marker of personal identity, as well as the need for a medium for social interaction. For example, an expectation as we age is decreased mobility and general deterioration in functioning, which themselves are possible contributors to alienation and deterioration. These and other challenges can create a strong need for patterns of stable behaviours, even if those behaviours, such as excessive alcohol consumption, have detrimental consequences (case study 1).

CASE STUDY 1

Mr B is 67 years old, a WWII veteran of the Polish Army, who came to Canada in 1946. Retired for two years, Mr B maintains his own home and is remarkably fit. However, his alcohol consumption, escalated since his retirement, has resulted in estrangement from his wife and two children. Since his wife left, Mr B goes to the local tavern for his main meal, and engages in alcohol consumption there, the norm in this environment. His family members, although witness to the negative consequences of his excess alcohol behaviour, are ambivalent about addressing his consumption behaviour. From their perspective, alcohol has strong associations with masculine and paternal qualities, and it would be an insult to their father's manhood to suggest that his alcohol consumption behaviour was negatively impacting on their lives. His beverage of choice is vodka, heavily imbibed in social situations, including with family. Mr B is not inhibited by public intoxication. This pattern is indicative of much of Eastern European consumption patterns for males.

Two years later, Mr B is visited by a home care worker. Apparently, one month earlier, Mr. B, unsteady after an evening at the tavern, stumbled on his front steps and fractured his ankle. This impaired him from visiting the tavern. Meals on Wheels now delivers meals to his home, and Mr B uses an alcohol delivery service. His children are finding it increasingly difficult to visit their father, as it is now painful to see him consuming alcohol alone in his home. The home care worker is concerned about Mr B's physical and social withdrawal from what little community involvement he had. The amount of alcohol consumed has not increased; however, the negative repercussions of his alcohol consumption are increasingly obvious due to his long consumption history combined with factors related to ageing. It is evident to the home care worker that Mr B has a strong relationship with his alcohol.

Sometimes more significant for an older person than for a younger person is the analgesic effect of alcohol. Physiology explains this. For an older person, perhaps due to metabolic changes that happen as we age, or perhaps due to lower water volume,[2] progressively less alcohol is needed to have the same effect. For an older person there is increased likelihood of chronic and acute health problems, and cognitive problems, possibly the result of long-term high alcohol consumption levels.[3] These chronic problems may also be responded to by using alcohol specifically for its analgesic and mood-altering effects.

Problematic consumption

Typology

Onset of problematic consumption has served as the basis for a typology of older adults with problematic consumption. Knowledge of the commencement of problematic consumption can have implications for identification of other problem issues, for treatment planning and for outcome expectations. Rosin and Glatt[4] developed the early- and late-onset typology. Graham *et al.*[5] described and expanded the number of types to three:

1 the early-onset was renamed chronic
2 late-onset was called reactive
3 where consumption was affected by cognitive and psychiatric problems.

The reactive group, Graham *et al.* suggest, is consuming in response to stressors of ageing (grief, retirement, relocation, health problems). Because the chronic group has a longer history of problematic consumption, they are more likely to have more physical, social and psychological complications,[5] and the consequences of long-term use are more visible than those for the reactive group with a shorter problematic consumption history. However, both the chronic and reactive groups are consuming in response to loneliness, isolation, boredom and poor self-esteem.

Graham *et al.*[5] found that treatment for the chronic group tended to focus on activities of daily living (ADL), while for the reactive group, grief counselling or retirement planning seemed to be the focus of treatment. In other words, ADL problems, and therefore interventions, are more likely in the chronic group than in the reactive group. (See 'Notes on activities of daily living', below).

The independent raters in Graham *et al's.* typology study[5] did not come to a consensus as to whether the third type, those whose consumption was affected by cognitive/psychiatric problems, was a subgroup of the chronic consumers. However, the experience of the author is that the recognition of the issues of cognitive and psychiatric factors has an impact on goal-setting, treatment and outcome expectations. A clear understanding of the interplay between cognitive impairment, psychiatric complications and alcohol consumption can reduce frustration due to expectations that are not realistic and lack of improvement in treatment.

Notes on activities of daily living (ADL)

The concept of ADL is a significant one when working with older adults. ADL include common self-care activities, such as dressing, personal hygiene, cooking and other primary activities. Although integral, yet often unnoticed, ADLs must be performed successfully so that the older adult can live safely, and independently, in the community.

A thorough assessment will form the basis for an intervention aimed at restoration of functioning. Measurement is essential in any strategy for improving health status. Yet, general health measures have limited value in indicating the *functioning* level a person can or does achieve.[6]

Almost all scales include some combination of dressing, bathing, toileting, transfer and feeding. Bowel and bladder continence, mobility and wheelchair mobility also appear on some scales, and some factor in the time it takes to perform the task. Scores are usually based on the degree of independence. Scales can be designed for institutional settings, or for more independent and home settings. Since the choice of scale may influence the results, a registered occupational therapist should be consulted for the selection and for the interpretation of the results.

Instrumental ADL, or IADL, include a range of activities more complex than those needed for personal care. These items are more likely to be sensitive to mood and emotional health. For instance, the inability to cook one's meals may be related to emotional abilities as well as physical abilities.[6]

The important concept is systematic collection and analysis of commonly agreed upon ADL variables to allow for comparisons, goal setting, indication of progress and evaluation. Another practical strategy is to ensure that all members of a multidisciplinary team use the same definitions and that assessors are clearly instructed in the correct method to make ADL observations.

Safety is an issue that needs to be considered in an assessment. The **S**afety **A**ssessment of **F**unction and the **E**nvironment for **R**ehabilitation (SAFER) Tool is a screening tool which addresses the functional capabilities and the environmental safety of the elderly living in the community. It consists of 15 areas of concern. When completed, it provides clear directions for interventions.[7]

While the ADL assessment may be completed by individuals from numerous disciplines, some healthcare providers may need to refer identified problems to occupational therapists for further evaluation and treatment.[6]

Identification

Although it is important to address each case individually, generalities are necessary to condense and analyse findings. These findings suggest that the profiles of older adults differ from those of younger persons with problems related to substance use. These differences suggest that a discrete screening tool is needed for older adults. This can result in a treatment plan that is distinct from that for younger persons.

For the older person there is:[3,8]

- higher rate of cognitive deficits
- lower maximum alcohol consumption
- greater need to drink before breakfast
- higher proportion who want to stop drinking but cannot
- lower probability of job problems
- lower probability of problems with friends or neighbours
- lower probability of problems with police
- increased probability of acute or long-term problems.

The above comparative profile has significant implications for identification. For example, the justice system is less likely to be involved with an older person than with a younger person; there is increased likelihood for an older person to have a primary diagnosis that reflects cognitive pathology than for a younger person; the healthcare system is more likely to be involved with an older person than with a younger person. There is also indication that older persons can be more motivated to change than younger persons.[3]

There is discussion in the literature on barriers to identification and treatment.[9,10] These barriers include poor screening tools, lack of knowledge about identification, diagnosing and interventions, as well as attitudes about older adults and problematic alcohol consumption.

Significant efforts have been made to develop tools that assist with identification and intervention. Among them, two are described here.

- *Alternatives*[11] is a training package, containing a stand-alone video with intervention re-enactments, and five manuals of supportive material for an independent workshop on this subject. (Much of the *identification* and *intervention* material in this chapter is in presentation-ready form in *Alternatives*. For information on ordering *Alternatives*, see 'To learn more', p. 256.)
- Modification of a self-administered screening instrument has resulted in the *MAST-G*,[12] with reportedly more effectiveness than the unaltered version in identifying problematic alcohol consumption. (See Appendix 8.1, p. 92, for a full version of the *MAST-G*.) Examples of questions that are specific to an older adult's situation include:
  - Have you increased your drinking after experiencing a loss in your life?
  - Does alcohol make you sleepy so that you often fall asleep in your chair?

Who identifies? Those who are likely to identify tend to be those who are visiting the home – service providers, staff of seniors' housing, volunteers and family members. In the community, emergency department and other hospital staff are also in a position to identify when confronted with the acute and chronic consequences of problematic alcohol consumption.

Behavioural, verbal and visual indicators[13]

Behavioural indicators that can assist identification include:

- multiple/expired medication use
- doctor/pharmacy shopping

- alcohol consumption while on medication
- excessive alcohol consumption
- excessive use of mints or perfume
- thinking difficulties (confusion, forgetfulness)
- defensiveness when asked to clarify consumption patterns
- chair *nesting*, with TV tray, remote, ashtray, cigarettes and alcohol (perhaps hidden) nearby
- neglect of home and or bills
- appearance of depressive affect
- erratic sleep patterns
- social withdrawal
- impaired coordination.

Verbal indicators include:

- substance-use problem
- vague health problems, like headaches or flu-like symptoms
- memory lapses or blackouts
- loneliness and helplessness
- loss of sex drive, complaints of impotence
- family history of drug problems
- history of physical abuse
- persistent financial difficulties.

Visual (physical appearance) indicators include:

- poor hygiene
- bruising, especially at furniture height. (Asking a client to remove his cap indoors may reveal subcutaneous contusions or lacerations on the forehead.)
- alcohol odour on breath, clothes or in the air
- weight gain or loss
- slurred speech
- broken blood vessels on the face
- fatigue
- chronic gastric problems
- flu-like symptoms
- skin changes
- blackouts
- oedema
- tremors.

Self-assessment question

The box below contains a case description. When reading it, select the indicators of a substance-use problem as listed above, or your own, that would indicate problems that are related to substance use. Check your list against the author's (see 'Answers to self-assessment questions', p. 233).

CASE STUDY 2

Mr H, aged 62, took early retirement and is living at home with his wife, Anne. In the last few years he has suffered increased memory loss and disorientation. Most recently, Mr H fractured his ankle when he stumbled on the stairs. A home assessment was offered to Anne when she described these issues with her physician. Because of Mr H's limited mobility, a home visiting nurse was arranged.

The nurse arrived at 10 a.m. and was greeted by Anne. Anne introduced her to Mr H, who was sitting in his recliner, bandaged foot up, watching television. The remote was on the table beside him. Also on the table were an untouched sandwich and a large beverage tumbler. There was an odour of alcohol in the area of the room where Mr H was sitting. There was a cut on Mr H's forehead. His sweater had large holes in the elbow. Although there were indications from Anne that Mr H wasn't eating well, such as weight loss, his abdomen seemed swollen.

Mr H was pleasant enough, and engaged easily in conversation about the weather. When asked whether he watched the hockey play-offs last night, he agreed then focused on legendary hockey greats of the 1940s. His speech was slow and slurred. When Anne suggested he turn the TV down, Mr H had obvious difficulty even picking up the remote; it was Anne who followed through with pushing the appropriate button. The nurse continued the discussion of the hockey legends, but it was obvious that Mr H had lost that train of thought.

When the nurse asked about his health, Mr H said he felt 'punk' all the time, and couldn't be more definitive. When asked about how much alcohol he consumed on an average day, Mr H dismissed the suggestion that alcohol consumption was causing any problems, seemed to have no memory of how much he was consuming, and, raising his voice, said 'So, what's the difference anyway?'

Because there are symptoms of ageing that can mimic alcohol consumption problems, and vice versa, there is a strong need for thorough assessment to avoid both a misdiagnosis and a missed opportunity to intervene. Following is a list of signs that can be attributed to ageing or to a substance-use problem:[13]

- confusion
- depression/disorientation
- unsteady gait/falls
- short-term memory loss
- loss of interest in activities
- social isolation
- tremors
- irregular heart rate
- poor appetite
- stomach complaints.

Treatment

Resource material on addiction treatment for older persons is limited compared to that for women and youth. Significant efforts to increase the literature base began in earnest in the 1970s. Gurnack[14] has made a comprehensive review of early and more contemporary literature on this issue. More recent approaches to treatment came from Saunders[15] and her development of the Community Older Persons Alcohol (COPA) addiction treatment programme, a home-visiting harm reduction approach after which several treatment programmes have been modelled.

Addiction-specific treatment has historically been a place where a person goes for treatment, whether it is offered within the practice of a therapist or family doctor or at an addiction-specific residential or day-treatment programme. It is a criterion of treatment that a person goes to the setting. For that to happen requires either recognition of a problem or external pressure to change. Many persons would not or could not meet these criteria. Presently recognised barriers include child-care commitments, language or culture, distance, mobility impairment or psychological impairment, whether these barriers are the causes or the effects of the substance use.

With increased knowledge and research on this issue, there are increasing numbers of treatment programmes for older persons, with the following common elements:[13]

- outreach or home visiting
- optimal medical care
- counselling and practical problem solving
- targeting improved functioning versus abstinence from alcohol
- addressing use of leisure time

- improved socialising skills
- resolving ADL. This is a basic concern of home-visiting services, because the assumption cannot be made that a person is mobile enough to come to treatment. ADL extend to social interactions, such as using the telephone, banking services, completing applications, making and keeping appointments, shopping, cooking and self-care.

Roles of the worker and of the organisation

The roles of the worker have been categorised as follows:

- home visiting
- rapport building
- assessment and treatment planning and implementing
- ongoing support
- problem resolution
- crises managing
- advocating.

Before elaborating further on these roles of the worker, it is critical to examine the role of the organisation. For without organisational support, demonstrated by appropriately allocated resources, it becomes frustrating and almost impossible for the worker to provide the needed services. In fact, although it may appear initially as if additional resources are needed to resolve the identified issues, a more comprehensive examination of the resources provided by home support services to an older person with substance use problems may reveal a reduction in overall service allocation. This reduction can be expected over the long term with improved functioning, increased independence, health and financial stability.

The roles of the worker are a hybrid between those of a visiting service provider with a geriatric perspective and an addiction worker. *Home visiting* to assist with the assessment of ADL, accommodation, accessibility and impact of consumption can have significant advantages, particularly for the first few visits. Accessibility and attendance is addressed; functioning with the activities of daily living can be observed; safety and social supports can be assessed; information provided verbally by the client can be collaborated through observations.

After obtaining information from the home visit and after establishing *rapport*, office visits can be considered. With the time it takes a client to commute to and from the office, visits can preclude alcohol consumption.

The *development of rapport* is critical for ongoing involvement. One of the barriers to establishing rapport is insistence that the focus of discussion be on substance use. It is common that in the worker's and client's perspective there are other issues that need more immediate attention. Examples might be medical care, nutritional needs or community services. Offering assistance for these issues will often strengthen the bond between worker and client. And therein lies the basis for *rapport-building* and subsequent visits. There will be opportunities, sometimes within the first visit, to point out the relationship between these issues and consumption levels. *Ongoing support* that results in the demonstration of *problem resolution*, sometimes with decreased consumption, will solidify the relationship and be the basis for ongoing consumption pattern changes.

For people living in the community who are vulnerable or frail, there is more likelihood of crises that must be addressed before agenda items. Acute medical complications, falls and exploitation are examples. *Crisis management* then becomes a role of the worker.

Assessment, treatment plan and implementation are grouped together for logistic and philosophical reasons. The purpose of the *assessment* is to develop a *treatment plan* that will attempt to resolve the identified issues. For example, if there is a problem with financial management, and a savings bank account has not been established because of loss of required identification documents, then the treatment plan would include obtaining the required documentation to open the account as part of the plan to address financial management. The *implementation* of this plan becomes an additional role of the worker. So often, issues are identified in the assessment but then left unresolved. Again, organisational support is required to pursue this strategy.

With a potentially vulnerable and frail population, there can often be a mismatch with community services. Some community services and resources understandably require a basic level of sophistication, including self-identification and articulation of needs. Assisting in performing these tasks, and *advocating* on behalf of the client to achieve a better match between the services and the client, become additional roles of the worker.

Assessment

As is the case for the roles of the worker, the categories for assessment are a hybrid between a geriatric home assessment, with its emphasis on ADL, and a bio/psycho/socio/spiritual addiction assessment. Assessments of ADL require often several home visits, and will usually determine the amount of time needed for assessments. In addition, it is not unusual for identified crises or critically important interventions to supersede the scheduled attempts to obtain the assessment.

Assessment data may fall into the following categories:

- substance use
- physical–emotional–mental health conditions
- relationships
- leisure and spiritual activities
- accommodation
- ADL.

Space will not allow for elaboration on all categories, most of which are addressed in the literature on ADL assessments. With respect to the substance use issue, however, clarification will be provided.

Substance use

It has been noted in the literature on counselling[16] that the manner in which a question is presented can have an impact on the response. Miller states that 'individuals in precontemplation about a problem behaviour … are not even thinking about changing that behaviour. In fact, they may not see the behaviour as a problem'.[17] With a client who is *precontemplative,* the following are suggestions for phrasing questions:[13]

- assume the substance is used – normalise consumption; be non-judgemental
- determine consumption history pattern, period of abstinence, triggers for relapsing and their meanings
- use their terms and value system
- ask for clarification if there are discrepancies.

Termination guidelines

The establishment of a potentially long-term relationship is a logistical requirement because many of the issues will take time to address. It is also an ethical requirement: because of increasing frailty and vulnerability that result from ageing and from long-term problematic consumption, there is increased likelihood of exploitation and of a history of prematurely terminated relationships. To terminate the client–worker relationship too soon, before other supports or skill-sets are established, can be antitherapeutic. The essence of treatment is also a strategy to prepare for termination, assisting the client with the development of positive relationships with the community, including family members if appropriate. This in turn decreases dependence on the worker upon appropriate termination.

As simplistic as the above sounds, it is necessary for the worker to be grounded in reality. There are many people who have no positive supports beyond the service provided by this worker. And for those, while continuing to work towards establishing other positive supports, maintaining the relationship is the only ethical choice. It must also be realised that termination is sometimes the result of death of the client. This is an unusual outcome within the addictions service sector, but is not unusual within the realm of service provision for older or frail individuals. These outcomes, both *long-term relationships* with clients who do not otherwise have significant supports, and *death*, have implications for evaluation.

Notes on evaluation

Admitting one has a problem is not the goal of treatment in a client-centred programme for older persons – the client may never admit a problem and may die first. Instead, working with the client to improve functioning, and to integrate with positive supports, family, individuals and community resources, is the ultimate goal. Concurrent with this, and a requirement for this goal, may be reduced problematic consumption of substances.

The above-discussed treatment goals have implications for evaluation. For instance, lengthy stay in treatment may skew a costing analysis when compared with other addiction treatment programmes for younger persons that are not outreach in nature. Death of a client may also skew the results. Clients need not admit nor recognise that they have a problem with substances, even though significant functional improvement, and even decreased consumption, may be evident.

One suggested method to address these issues in evaluation is to develop a list of the desired outcomes. An example of this may look like:

- Assist client to make and attend a medical appointment to determine reason for pain when urinating.
- Assist client to replace identification stolen when mugged while intoxicated.
- Assist client to contact daughter to determine her well-being.
- Support client to attend a socialising group in the community.
- Arrange for meals to be delivered.

However, a difficulty with this approach to evaluation (a credit to the worker's skill) is that additional issues are identified during treatment. For instance, in the case above, terminal cancer as well as bladder infection was identified. There was significant suspicion that it was not a *mugger* but the daughter who had stolen, and was continuing to steal her mother's money. Moreover, the conditions for delivery of the meals required that the client be home to receive the delivery, jeopardising the possibility of attending the socialising group. This then resulted in an amended and enhanced list of objectives to be addressed by the worker. By advocating and addressing each issue, significant developments were made by the worker to improve the client's quality of life:

• the meal delivery service amended its condition, allowing for attendance at the socialising group
• the daughter was charged with fraud
• a comprehensive palliative care plan was developed
• alcohol consumption decreased dramatically to a non-problematic level
• urinary pain was arrested.

However, at termination, and time of death, there were more issues than were presented at intake.

Another potential outcome anomaly may be that clients are not home for their scheduled visits. For clients who may have a history of not leaving their homes, this can be interpreted as an indication that they are reintegrating into their community in a positive fashion again. On the other hand, memory impairment may be such that keeping appointments is not an expectation. Both of these outcomes must be analysed in context.

Graham[9] identifies additional issues in evaluation: the lack of valid measures of problematic substance consumption among older persons; the lack of valid measures for monitoring other life areas; the individualised and flexible nature of the treatment, with no standard length of stay and no standard intervention. Due to a large part to Graham's efforts in this area, it is increasingly recognised that the traditional measures of success – admitting a problem, followed by abstinence – need to be re-examined.

Concurrent issues to investigate

Gambling

The many changes and losses in the lives of seniors result in a special vulnerability to the risks presented by gambling.[18] These changes and losses include:

• loneliness resulting from the loss of a spouse, family members or special friends

- retirement and a feeling of loss of self-esteem that sometimes comes with it
- moves from the familiar surrounding of the family home to smaller apartments
- anxiety over changes in health
- concern for financial security
- feelings of isolation and loneliness that may come from reduced social contacts and community involvement.

With many of these changes and losses, seniors look for something to fill the void. Gambling can become an exciting alternative. There are added risks for seniors. Often marketing and incentives from gaming establishments are targeted at seniors. Others, including professionals, may suggest and encourage gambling activities such as casino excursions and bingo. Increasing sensitivity to addressing and preventing problematic gambling behaviours, and advocating for appropriate treatment for seniors with gambling problems, are activities that can result in change.

Home detoxification

'Home detoxification', or community-based withdrawal management, is a service that has the potential to reduce episodes of in-patient care, with its inherent high costs and secondary problems of label attachment and possible stigmatisation. Excellent resource material on 'home detoxification' is available.[19]

Home detoxification is a logical service to address mobility limitations of the older adult. In Toronto, the COPA addiction treatment programme for older adults is providing community-based withdrawal management services for this population. The protocol used is a modification of that developed by Stockwell[20] for his project for the general population in Exeter, England. For more information on community withdrawal management for the older person, contact the author.[21]

Elder abuse

The proportion of frail elderly is increasing, as is the need for caregivers. Alcohol-related problems can only exacerbate existing stress on the caregivers. There is evidence that elder abuse will increase due to: fewer adult offspring to share the care of the growing number of frail elderly; increasing number of caregivers who are elderly children; and increasing number of females unavailable as caregivers because of engagement in other work.[22] Screening for, treating and preventing elder abuse become important roles for the worker.

Consultation to professional and non-professional caregivers

Efforts to increase the responsiveness of existing addiction treatment facilities to the needs of older persons who can access a facility, include training of addiction personnel, consultation on programme design and resource allocation. Discussion around training material has been provided earlier. In addition, work has been done around the development of a questionnaire to address systemic barriers.[23] To respond to these questions, an organisational perspective is needed that will increase awareness regarding the allocation of organisational resources to the needs of the older adults.

Clinical consultation services, when one specific client's situation is discussed with professionals and others who are caring for them is offered in Toronto by telephone. The evaluation of this service[24] suggests that users are pleased with its convenience and accessibility, and find it very helpful to obtain guidance and support from a professional who is dedicated to the treatment of substance use and older persons.

Conclusion

The relationship between alcohol use and older adults has received little attention until recently. The dearth of knowledge on this issue, coupled with the potential complications when a worker confronts this situation, can create the illusion that the task of providing treatment is formidable. However, it is only an illusion, for repeatedly, with commitment and knowledge, workers can make a difference in the lives of older adults who have problems related to substance use. An attitude of openness and respect can create the atmosphere for meaningful interactions, mutual growth and sharing. It is hoped that the issues presented above provide stimulation to pursue this rewarding work, and to research the many areas that yet are unexplored.

To develop your knowledge in this area, see 'To learn more', pp. 256–7.

The Community Older Persons Alcohol Program (COPA) has legally changed its name to Community Outreach Programs in Addiction (COPA).

The Addiction Research Foundation has merged with three other institutions to become the Center for Addiction and Mental Health.

Self-assessment question

This chapter was designed as an introduction to the issue of older persons and substance use. What additional steps can you take to enhance your ability to further address this issue? Compare your ideas with those of the author in 'Answers to self-assessment questions – Chapter 8', pp. 234–5.

Appendix 8.1 Michigan Alcoholism Screening Test – Geriatric Version (MAST-G)

DIRECTIONS: The following is a list of questions about your past and present drinking habits. Please answer yes or no to each question by marking the line next to the question. When you are finished answering the questions, please add up how many 'yes' responses you checked and put that number in the space provided at the end.

		YES	NO
1	After drinking, have you ever noticed an increase in your heart rate or beating in your chest?		
2	When talking to others, do you ever underestimate how much you actually drank?		
3	Does alcohol make you sleepy so that you often fall asleep in your chair?		
4	After a few drinks, have you sometimes not eaten or been able to skip a meal because you didn't feel hungry?		
5	Does having a few drinks help you decrease your shakiness or tremors?		
6	Does alcohol sometimes make it hard for you to remember parts of the day or night?		
7	Do you have rules for yourself that you won't drink before a certain time of the day?		
8	Have you lost interest in hobbies or activities you used to enjoy?		
9	When you wake up in the morning, do you ever have trouble remembering part of the night before?		
10	Does having a drink help you sleep?		
11	Do you hide your alcohol bottles from family members?		
12	After a social gathering, have you ever felt embarrassed because you drank too much?		
13	Have you ever been concerned that drinking might be harmful to your health?		
14	Do you like to end an evening with a nightcap?		
15	Did you find your drinking increased after someone close to you died?		
	In general, would you prefer to have a few drinks at home rather than go out to social events?		
16	Are you drinking more now than in the past?		
17	Do you usually take a drink to relax or calm your nerves?		
18	Do you drink to take your mind off your problems?		
19	Have you ever increased your drinking after experiencing a loss in your life?		
20	Do you sometimes drive when you have had too much to drink?		
21	Has a doctor or nurse ever said they were worried or concerned about your drinking?		
22	Have you ever made rules to manage your drinking?		
23	When you feel lonely, does having a drink help?		

Total 'yes' responses =

Scoring: 5 or more 'yes' responses is indicative of an alcohol problem.

For further information, contact Frederic Blow, PhD, at University of Michigan Alcohol Research Centre, 400 East Eisenhower Parkway, Suite 2A, Ann Arbor, MI 4810 5-3318, USA. Tel: (734) 9987952.

CHAPTER 9

Mental health and mental illness

Paul Clenaghan

Pre-reading exercise

Before reading this chapter:

1 Refer to a mental health textbook on common mental health problems and, in particular, psychosis (for example, Hilgard, Atkinson and Atkinson (1996) Abnormal psychology. In *Introduction to Psychology* (12th edn), published by Harcourt Brace Jovanovich).
2 Consider some of the common myths about substance use and mental illness.
3 Consider some of the following questions.

- What are your beliefs about the association between mental illness and substance use?
- What are some of the commonly held beliefs about mental illness and substance use?
- Why do people use alcohol?
- Why do you or your friends use alcohol?
- Do you or your friends use alcohol in an attempt to improve your mental health or social interactions?
- Do you or your friends suffer mental health problems from using alcohol?
- How is the treatment of someone with alcohol problems and mental illness managed in our current health systems?
- How could the treatment be improved?

Introduction

> *'People with a mental illness are at a higher risk of developing problematic alcohol use. People with problematic alcohol use are at a higher risk of developing a mental illness.'*[1]

The relationship between alcohol use and mental illness is complex and cannot be ignored. Alcohol use may mask symptoms of a mental illness, or indeed symptoms of a mental illness may be a temporary effect of alcohol use.

In order to effectively treat people who have both a mental illness and a problem with alcohol use, it is necessary to explore the area that you are less familiar with (for most readers this is mental illness), and then integrate this knowledge with the skills you already possess.

This chapter focuses on problematic alcohol use and what is often referred to as the major mental illnesses (such as schizophrenia and bipolar affective disorder). This group of mental illnesses is considered to have the highest incidence of problematic alcohol use, though the services and models of treatment discussed are also applicable to depression, anxiety and many other mental illnesses. Similarly, the treatment related to problems with alcohol use will be applicable to other drug use (such as cannabis). See Appendix 9.1 for information on the nature of psychosis.[2]

Key discussion points include:

- what is the relationship between mental illness and alcohol use?
- why do people with mental illness use alcohol?
- types of 'dual disorder'
- the impact of mental illness and alcohol use
- alcohol and suicide
- overcoming barriers to effective treatment
- what is the treatment of psychosis?
- recommended treatment for people with mental illness and problematic alcohol use.

The association between mental illness and alcohol use

It is widely believed that alcohol use:

- precipitates mental illness
- exacerbates symptoms of mental illness
- reduces or exaggerates the effects of psychotropic medication (e.g. antipsychosis medication)
- reduces the person's compliance with treatment.

The complexity of the relationship has been described in three ways:[1]

1 mental illness that causes alcohol use
2 mental illness that is a result of alcohol use
3 chance associations.

It has frequently been found that approximately half of all persons who experience psychosis also suffer from co-occurring problematic drug or alcohol use:[3–11]

- American epidemiological studies have indicated prevalence rates for significant problems with alcohol use and other drug use of around 7% *in the general population.*
- People with a history *of major depression or anxiety have double the risk.*
- Approximately *50% of young people with schizophrenia or bipolar affective disorder* are likely to have a significant problem with alcohol or other drugs.

Why people with mental illness use alcohol

There are several theories about the reasons why people with a mental illness use alcohol:

- for the same reasons other people in the community use alcohol
- as an attempt to alleviate the symptoms of mental illness
- to reduce side-effects of medication.

Theory 1: For the same reasons other people in the community use alcohol

People with a mental illness use alcohol for many of the same reasons as other people in the community. Box 9.1 lists some of these reasons.

Box 9.1 Reasons why people use alcohol[1]

- to change or elevate mood
- to reduce anxiety
- to increase confidence
- for socialisation
- because of peer-group pressure
- to engage in a ceremony or ritual
- for avoidance or escape
- for an experience of ecstasy or bliss

- for a spiritual experience
- to increase motivation, energy and wakefulness
- to aid creativity
- for recreation
- to sleep
- for experimentation or exploration
- to rebel or to attract attention
- to reduce self-consciousness
- to reduce pain
- for excitement or thrills

Case examples

1 Sarah is an 18-year-old who describes herself as very shy. She experiences anxiety and has panic attacks. Sarah drinks alcohol at weekends – this helps her self-confidence and ability to socialise.
2 Thomas is a 63-year-old author. Thomas has mood swings and has been diagnosed as having a bipolar affective disorder. Thomas drinks alcohol when he is writing and believes this improves his creativity.

Theory 2: As an attempt to alleviate the symptoms of mental illness

People with a mental illness could have even greater motivation to improve the areas detailed in Box 9.1 since mental illness frequently has a significant impact on these aspects of their lives. For example, the residual symptoms of schizophrenia can include dysphoria, low motivation and energy level, anxiety, a desire for socialisation and fun.[12] People with schizophrenia report that alcohol can help with anxiety, dysphoria and insomnia.[13]

Case examples

3 John is a 21-year-old man who has schizophrenia. He experiences auditory hallucinations (voices) and has become more withdrawn over the last two years. John has not worked for the past two years and has little contact with people apart from his family. John has discovered that drinking alcohol gives him temporary relief from the voices: 'It seems to drown the voices out or sometimes it helps me to handle the voices.' John also knows that he interacts and socialises better with people when

he has had several drinks. John recognises that the next day he may feel worse but the temporary relief, he believes, is worth it.

4 George is a 55-year-old man who has recently lost his job (redundancy). George's wife died 10 months ago and he is still grieving. George finds it difficult to sleep, he has lost his appetite and most of the time feels miserable. George has very few close friends. George goes to the pub every evening and has developed friendships with some of the 'regulars'. He finds that he is able to sleep after drinking several beers. Each day George feels more depressed and finds his main relief or escape from this depression can be found in the pub.

Theory 3: To reduce side-effects of medication

It is common for people who are treated with antipsychosis medication to experience unpleasant side-effects. Some people report feeling empty, joyless, inactive and unimaginative (the opposite of some of the list in Box 9.1). People who have schizophrenia and take antipsychosis medication sometimes use alcohol to regain the self that is subdued by medication.[1]

Some people see their drug or alcohol use as a solution to the problems associated with their mental illness or to problems associated with the medication that is prescribed for their mental illness.

Recommendation: Health professionals are able to determine treatment interventions based on why the drugs or alcohol are being used and treat the underlying problem as opposed to identifying drug or alcohol use as 'the problem'.

Types of mental illness and alcohol use

People who have both a mental illness and problematic alcohol use are a diverse group. They have varying degrees of disability associated with their varying experiences of these dual problems. The experience of having both a mental illness and problematic alcohol use is not static. A person may move through various phases in their life, at one time requiring medication or detoxification, at another time requiring counselling and support.

As Figure 9.1 illustrates, any one person may be located at different points along the scale at different stages in their life and consequently require different types of treatment. Generally, it is the group in the centre for whom less service exists.

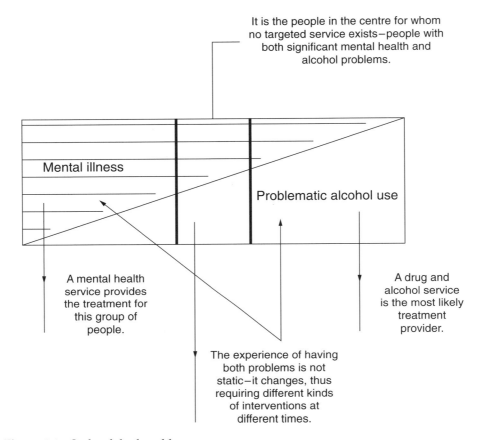

Figure 9.1 Scale of dual problems.

The impact of having a mental illness and problems with alcohol

As indicated above, people who experience these dual problems are a diverse group. They have a complex range of problems related to the mental illness, the effects of alcohol use on their lives, and the interaction between alcohol use and the mental illness. *Research indicates that rates of recovery for people with mental illness and problematic alcohol use are lower than that of people who have only one 'disorder'.*[1]

Studies report that alcohol use is associated with a variety of adverse consequences for people with schizophrenia, including:

- increase in hallucinations
- increase in delusions
- increase in paranoia
- increase in depressive symptoms
- increase in disruptive behaviour
- increase in housing instability and homelessness.[5, 6, 14–19]

A person often reports a benefit from using alcohol. However, the negative effects often occur not only at the time of use but also the next day or next week.

Alcohol, suicide and mental illness

Special mention is required regarding the relationship between alcohol, suicide and mental illness. Alcohol is frequently associated with suicidal behaviour, and is involved in 20–50% of suicide cases.[20] The involvement of alcohol can be viewed in two ways:

1 Alcohol, through its disinhibiting and depressant effects, can contribute to the decision to suicide, which is often impulsive.
2 Alcohol can be used for so-called 'Dutch courage' to facilitate the fatal action or to anaesthetise against the discomfort (physical and emotional) of suicide.

Furthermore, many people with long-term alcohol and other drug problems attempt suicide. For example, one study found that people with substance use problems accounted for up to 50% of suicidal deaths among 15–24 year-olds.[21]

The link between suicide and mental illness is well established and estimates indicate that young people with a mental illness are more than 10 times more likely to attempt suicide.[22] The combination of these two problems (alcohol and mental illness) emphasises the urgency of overcoming barriers to treatment and identifying effective treatment strategies.

Overcoming barriers to treatment

The group of people towards the centre of the scale of dual problems (see Figure 9.1) experience barriers to treatment due to deficiencies in the model of health service delivery.

Barrier 1: Separate systems

Despite the high incidence of these dual problems, few programmes provide the comprehensive services needed to address both problems simultaneously.

Recommendation: An integrated approach – people experience problems from mental illness and alcohol concurrently, therefore it seems logical that treatment should be concurrent. This approach demonstrates that both types of problems are present and both can be treated.

Barrier 2: Lack of education and training

Mental health services are provided by professionals with minimal training or experience in the treatment of problematic alcohol use. Similarly, drug and alcohol treatment services are provided by professionals with little ongoing training in mental health.

Recommendation: There is a need to improve education and training about the other system of care (i.e. improved education and training for mental health professionals about alcohol use and treatment, and training for drug and alcohol treatment providers about mental illness and treatment).

Many curricula require expanding to include specific topics related to these dual problems.

Barrier 3: Lack of tailored and flexible treatment

The people towards the centre of the scale of dual problems (see Figure 9.1) generally have poorer access to treatment services or may report that the treatment programme does not fit with their range of problems (or their understanding of their problems). For many people the existing treatment services will be appropriate. For others, a more flexible and tailored treatment programme is required (e.g. particularly people who need a comprehensive range of services, a longer period of treatment or find it extremely difficult to commit to abstinence).

Recommendations:
1 Harm minimisation – The goal of harm minimisation is to enable people to make realistic choices about their future alcohol use. The approach of harm minimisation is particularly crucial for people who have multiple problems and few positive aspects to their lives and for whom there may be little incentive to achieve a goal of abstinence.[1]

2 Comprehensive – A holistic and comprehensive approach means that mental illness and problematic alcohol use symptoms cannot be viewed in isolation from each other. To provide adequate treatment, problems must be addressed on a number of levels.

3 Longitudinal – There is sometimes a need for a longitudinal perspective in viewing people with these dual problems. Treatment may need to occur continuously over years rather than episodically or during crises.

4 Hope – People with these dual problems and their families and friends are particularly likely to become discouraged and it is crucial that health professionals demonstrate optimism to clients and families. The need for a longitudinal perspective and optimism in viewing serious mental illnesses, such as schizophrenia, applies equally to problematic drug or alcohol use.

5 Basic needs first – The most effective treatment is achieved when basic needs are met and a person is well engaged with the treatment provider and treatment programme. A person who is hungry and homeless is less likely to care what a counsellor says about alcohol and mental health treatment than someone who has accommodation and feels safe and secure. Safety, housing and financial needs often require addressing at an early stage of treatment.

Treatment issues

For some readers it may be necessary to review the treatment recommendations of mental illnesses (such as psychosis) prior to reading the recommendations for treatment of mental illness and problematic alcohol use. A basic textbook on mental illness will provide this information, however some of the principles will be identified here.

In order to effectively treat people who have both a mental illness and a problem with alcohol use it is necessary to explore the area that you are less familiar with and then integrate this knowledge with the skills you already possess.

The treatment of psychosis

See Appendix 9.1 for information on what psychosis is.

Biological interventions
Antipsychosis medication is an essential starting point for treatment.

Psychological interventions
There is a vast range of psychological interventions. The best context for care (of the person with an acute episode of psychosis) is one of empathy and concern for the distress of the person and their family.

Box 9.2 How should I (a family member) relate to the person who is experiencing psychosis?

- Be yourself.
- Gain information and understand that the person may be behaving and talking differently due to the symptoms and or drug and alcohol misuse.
- Understand that symptoms of psychosis are stressful for everyone and that you may have a range of feelings – shock, fear, sadness, anger, frustration, despair.
- Talking to other people will help you to deal with these feelings. Believe a person will recover – even if it takes time. Be patient.
- Try not to take it personally if a person says hurtful words to you when they are unwell.
- When a person has acute symptoms of psychosis (or is under the influence of drugs or alcohol) they may be fixed in their beliefs and ideas. Do not become involved in a long disagreement, but listen with interest to gain an understanding of their current reality – to show sympathy and for future reference, to discuss when they are better.
- Take care of yourself. It is a balance between care and concern and not getting too run down yourself.

During an acute episode of psychosis the person's family needs information on how to relate to the person (Box 9.2)

Education acute phase
The initial aim is to minimise anxiety and confusion. During the acute phase, information should be simple, clear, concise and relevant (see Boxes 9.2 and 9.3).

Box 9.3 Examples of clear and concise information required

- Appropriate medication usually reduces symptoms of psychosis.
- No one is to blame for the illness – families do not cause psychosis.
- Symptoms of recent onset which are preceded by a severe stressor usually resolve, but may occur at a later date.
- It is important to minimise stress and stimulation during the acute episode.

Education post acute phase

The main goals of education are:

- to facilitate an understanding of the illness and its management by providing information on:
  - the nature of the illness
  - the importance of medication and associated issues, including avoidance of alcohol and other drugs
  - recognising and acting upon early warning signs of relapse
  - identifying and managing environmental stressors
  - identifying and developing social supports
- to recognise relapse triggers – the combination of stress and a vulnerability to stress are triggers for relapse
- to help the person and carers take an active role in the management of the illness
- to develop a therapeutic alliance and promote engagement in further psychological and social interventions
- to enable further assessment of current impairment, disability and handicap, and of goals or assets such as problem-solving skills or other effective coping strategies.

Comment: It is vital to recognise that diagnosis is often unclear where there is drug or alcohol use, particularly if the person is experiencing the first episode of psychosis. The diagnosis of schizophrenia cannot be made unless symptoms persist for a set period of time. The education should therefore stress the uncertainty of the diagnosis and the course or prognosis of the disorder.

Social interventions

The provision of practical assistance with social difficulties and structured problem solving is important (e.g. housing and financial problems, employment, legal problems including possible disputes over involuntary admission).[3]

The four stages of treatment for people with a mental illness and problems with alcohol

The recommendations for overcoming barriers to treatment identify crucial principles of treatment, including:

- an integrated approach
- improved education for treatment providers
- harm minimisation

- a comprehensive approach
- a longitudinal perspective
- hope
- meeting basic needs first.

The treatments of mental health problems include:

- biological interventions
- psychological interventions
- educational interventions
- social interventions.

The treatments of alcohol problems are discussed elsewhere in this book.

It is crucial to integrate all these principles and programmes into one comprehensive and flexible treatment programme which consists of four stages.[3]

1 engagement
2 persuasion
3 active treatment
4 relapse prevention.

Engagement

A person must be attracted to a treatment programme. This attraction may be helped by providing a range of useful and non-threatening services (e.g. assistance with housing, food and clothing; healthcare; provision of legal advice or referral; social and vocational opportunities).

The engagement stage is also the time during which a relationship is established with the therapist. If the person learns to trust and like the therapist, and believes the therapist is acting in their best interests, the person may become more interested in the notion of change.

During the engagement stage it is important not to make strong demands on the person to stop or reduce alcohol use, although it is acceptable for the therapist to indicate their disapproval of excessive alcohol intake. The engagement stage needs to be alluring and non-threatening. This phase may take a long time to develop to the point where stage 2 can be implemented.

Persuasion

The aim here is to help the person realise that they have a problem related to alcohol and to encourage the person to do something about this problem. Unfortunately, denial of the problem is a very strong defence mechanism and some people with a mental illness may find it particularly difficult to assess and alter their beliefs. Thought disorder, suspiciousness and depression may all influence the person's ability to adopt a new and more objective viewpoint. The persuasion stage of a treatment programme can be very challenging for the therapist. The following guidelines may be useful for persuading the person to accept help.

- Express concern for the person's well-being.
- Provide education – A person may not realise how the alcohol is affecting their mental health. Information may include:
  - the effects of alcohol on the body and on mental illness
  - highlighting other negative effects of alcohol (e.g. trouble with the police, social and relationship problems, lack of money)
  - discussing positive and negative effects of using alcohol
  - discussing problems in a person's life that may be making them turn to alcohol
  - indicating ways of improving life without alcohol
  - talking about what is involved in dealing with alcohol problems
  - encouraging attendance at group meetings for people with similar problems (if such meetings can be arranged).
- Discuss with others – Other people who have had similar problems and have coped well may be a resource of support and advice.
- Prepare for 'two steps forward and one step back' – If a person accepts assistance it is important that they realise that support and respect will not be withdrawn if early relapses occur. Relapses are to be expected as a minor setback, not as a failure.

Active treatment
Once the person has decided that they want to give up alcohol, the active treatment stage may begin. A thorough assessment is required, followed by an individually tailored treatment plan, devised ideally in conjunction with the person and their family.

- Assessment – The person will need an assessment of their physical, mental and social well-being:
  - frequency and quantity of alcohol use
  - other substances used
  - why the person is using alcohol
  - other co-existing problems that may be contributing to the alcohol use that may require treatment (e.g. physical illnesses, anxiety)
  - cues that trigger alcohol use
  - new skills that the person will need to acquire.
- Encourage substitute behaviours or environments – If the alcohol use is to be eliminated, alternative behaviours will have to be substituted for those that are presently associated with alcohol use:

- changes to peer group
- changes to recreational activities
- changing environments associated with alcohol (e.g. stop going to the pub)
- talking to family, friends, therapist about day-to-day problems rather than turning to alcohol
- rewarding periods of abstinence.

- Skills training – The person may require retraining of personal, vocational or social skills such as problem solving, goal planning, communication skills, job skills, assertiveness training.
- Support – Regular attention and praise for all efforts will be important motivators. Support and encouragement from family and friends will also be extremely beneficial.
- Monitoring – Symptoms and signs of relapse can be monitored (sometimes Breathalyser and urine tests are appropriate). Satisfactory test results can provide extra opportunity for praise and feedback.

Relapse prevention

Once a person has been alcohol-free for six months to a year, they graduate to the relapse prevention stage. During this stage the person will require ongoing contact and support from a therapist, family and friends. Success needs to be highlighted and praised. Occasional monitoring can be used.

It will be useful for the person and therapist to discuss how the person might feel if relapse occurs, and what action could be taken in such a situation.

Summary

People who have a mental illness and problems with alcohol are a diverse group and each person will have unique needs. These unique needs can diverge from traditional treatment models. This group of people have difficulties in many areas of treatment: accessing treatment programmes, entering into a treatment programme, assessment and review, support, community living, supported accommodation, and appropriate treatment and medications. The points to note are:

- People with a mental illness are at a higher risk of developing problematic alcohol use.
- People with problematic alcohol use are at a higher risk of developing a mental illness.
- There is a vast range of associations between mental illness and alcohol use.

- The combination of mental illness and problems with alcohol is generally more disabling than having a mental illness alone (or a problem with alcohol).
- There are extra barriers to treatment.
- Treatment needs to integrate principles from both mental health and drug and alcohol treatment services.
- Treatment needs to be flexible with a major emphasis on engagement. To develop your knowledge in this area, see 'To learn more', p. 258.

Self-assessment questions

1 Are people with a mental illness at a higher risk of developing problematic alcohol use? If so, why?
2 Are people with problematic alcohol use at a higher risk of developing a mental illness? If so, why?
3 What are some of the barriers to treatment for someone with both a mental illness and alcohol problems?
4 What would you recommend to overcome these treatment barriers?
5 What are the four groups of interventions that are used in the treatment of psychosis?
6 What are the stages of treatment for people with a mental illness and problems with alcohol?
7 What is the most challenging stage of treatment for people with a mental illness and problems with alcohol?
8 What are some of the common problems with the engagement stage of treatment and how would you overcome them?
9 How do you respond when a person drinks more alcohol (problematically) or their mental illness becomes worse?

Appendix 9.1 What is psychosis?

Psychosis describes conditions that affect the mind, causing some loss of contact with reality. It is most likely to occur in young adults. Around three out of every 100 people will experience a psychotic episode (it is more common than diabetes), and most people make a full recovery from psychosis.[2]

What are the symptoms of psychosis?

Psychosis may lead to changes in mood and thinking and to abnormal ideas, making it hard to understand how the person feels. It can be characterised by one or more of the following:

- *Confused thinking* – Everyday thoughts become jumbled or do not join up properly. Sentences are unclear and do not make sense. Thought processes seem to speed up or slow down.
- *False beliefs* – A person may hold a false belief, known as a delusion. The person is so convinced of their delusion that the most logical argument cannot make them change their mind. For example, someone may be convinced from the way cars are parked outside their house that they are being watched by the police.
- *Hallucinations* – The person sees, hears, feels, smells or tastes something that is not actually there. For example, they may hear voices that no one else can hear, or see things that aren't there.
- *Changed feelings* – A person may feel strange and cut off from the world with everything moving in slow motion. Mood swings are common and they may feel unusually excited or depressed. People's emotions may seem dampened – they feel less than they used to, or show less emotion to those around them.

Types of psychosis

- *Organic psychosis* – Sometimes psychotic symptoms may appear after a head injury or a physical injury which disrupts brain functioning, for example encephalitis, AIDS or a tumour. There are usually other symptoms present such as memory problems or confusion.
- *Brief reactive psychosis* – Psychotic symptoms may arise in response to a major stress in the person's life, such as a death or change of living circumstances. Symptoms can be severe, but the person makes a quick recovery.

- *Schizophrenia* – Schizophrenia refers to a psychotic illness in which the changes in behaviour or symptoms have been continuing for at least six months. The symptoms and length of the illness vary from person to person. It is important to remember that, contrary to popular belief, many people with schizophrenia lead happy and fulfilling lives and make a full recovery.
- *Schizophreniform disorder* – Symptoms of schizophrenia that have lasted for less than six months.
- *Bipolar (manic-depressive) disorder* – In bipolar disorder, psychosis appears as part of a more general disturbance in mood, in which mood is characterised by extreme highs (mania) or lows (depression). When psychotic symptoms are present, they tend to fit into the person's mood. For example, people who are depressed may hear voices telling them they should commit suicide; someone who is unusually excited or happy may believe they are special and can perform amazing feats.
- *Schizoaffective disorder* – This diagnosis is made when the person has concurrent or consecutive symptoms of both a mood disorder (mania or depression) and psychosis. In other words, the symptoms are not typical of a mood disorder or schizophrenia.
- *Psychotic depression* – Severe depression with psychotic symptoms, but without periods of mania or highs. This distinguishes the illness from bipolar disorder.
- *Drug-induced psychosis* – Use of, or withdrawal from, alcohol and drugs can be associated with the appearance of psychotic symptoms. Sometimes these symptoms will rapidly resolve as the effects of the drugs or alcohol wear off. In other cases the illness may last longer, but begins with drug-induced psychosis.

The causes of psychosis are not yet fully understood. There is some indication that psychosis is caused by a poorly understood combination of biological factors, which create a vulnerability to experiencing psychosis symptoms. These symptoms often emerge in response to stress, drug or alcohol use or social changes in such vulnerable individuals.

CHAPTER 10

Transcultural issues

Karin L Anseline

Pre-reading exercise

This exercise should take no more than 20 minutes. After reading the chapter, repeat the exercise to see if your understanding is the same or has improved.

1 Ask yourself, 'what cultures do I work with'?
2 How does your culture affect your view of other cultures?
3 List the differences between your culture and the cultures you work with.
4 List strategies you could use in assessing clients of different cultures.
5 List three cultures and how they view excessive alcohol use.
6 Consider whether the views above are the same for women.

It is important to be aware of cultural factors that may have a positive and or negative effect on our behaviour, and that of our clients. We need to be acutely aware of our own attitudes, values, behaviours and beliefs so that we can accept our client's own cultural reality. It is also important that we are not limited by our own world view of alcohol's place in society.

First we must understand what culture is. In general terms it has been described as 'the customs, beliefs, values, knowledge and skills that guide a people's behaviour along shared paths'.[1] However, a better description and one which allows us to consider how *we* live, and how the lives of others can at times can be so different, defines culture as:[2]

> *'our routine of sleeping, bathing, dressing, eating and getting to work. It is our household chores and the actions we perform on the job, the way we buy goods and services, write and mail a letter, take a taxi or board a bus, make a phone call, go to a movie or attend church. It is the way we greet friends or address a stranger, the admonitions and scolding we give our children and the way they regard what we consider good and bad manners, and even to a large extent what we consider right and wrong.*

All these and thousands of other ways of thinking, feeling and acting seem so natural and right that we may well wonder how else one could do it. But, to millions of other people in the world, every one of these acts would seem strange, awkward, incomprehensible, unnatural and wrong. These people would perform many, if not all, of the same acts but they would be done in different ways that to them would seem logical, natural and right.'

Taken together we see that we all have social signposts in our lives, things we would consider appropriate or inappropriate, and which may impinge on, or confirm, our most strongly held values to the extent that sanctions may apply to those who don't conform to our culture, beliefs or values.

The use of psychoactive substances amongst many people has been documented since earliest historical times. Each culture shares norms, beliefs and expectations that shape not only their drinking habits but the ways they may behave both while drinking and how they view personal and collective responsibility for the outcomes of drinking.[3]

Culture is not a genetic trait, rather it is an integral part of the environment, made and maintained by the members of each culture. It is learnt and passed on to each generation. It is shared, complex and dynamic. It combines a number of things which include customs, traditions, history and values. It is how people view their world and their place in it. It also determines what people value to preserve and pass on to future generations.

Some cultures have such strongly held views in relation to alcohol that no matter where they live, these views will be carried with them. This needs to be understood by those working with such clients.

This interplay between the person, their behaviour, culture and environment makes a point in highlighting that culture consists of many equally important ingredients. This requires that those working with clients using alcohol need to accept that people differ as individuals and as groups.

The early diffusion of culture came through invasion and colonisation. Indigenous people were particularly affected as there was often an attempt to break down indigenous cultures, which may have included forcibly removing children from their parents and a denigration of indigenous cultural values and traditions. This created generations of fragmented family life, and mental and physical health and other social problems. Today this legacy is viewed by both indigenous and non-indigenous communities as both a cause of alcohol and drug use, and a factor which can limit the effectiveness of intervention programmes.[4]

Alcohol problems have been seen to create devastating social, spiritual, and mental and physical health issues for many of the world's indigenous populations which include the Canadian Indians, Australian Aborigines, Hispanics and North American Indians. Many have taken the initiative to set up programmes of their own, which place a strong emphasis on the culture, and returning to their roots and reorienting of lifestyle. Indigenous communities need cooperation and respect so that their own culture can be used to attempt to deal with the problems that alcohol may bring.

Early migration was also a time of ethnic stereotyping, for example the drunk Irish and the Chinese opium dens, which was used to try and limit the influx of those groups to particular communities. It is amusing now to consider that coffee was banned in England (without success) by Charles II.

Today migration is in such large numbers that some persons may present with a combination of values in relation to alcohol that spring from their country of origin and their country of migration. This will be more prevalent amongst younger people, and those of second-generation families, as the families insist on maintaining tradition and the young people are more vulnerable to peer-group pressure and want to live like those in the host culture.

Therefore younger people's attitudes towards alcohol use will continuously change due to interaction between these cultures. This interaction will cause a change in the pattern of behaviour, either positively or negatively. One waits with interest to see the effects of the European Economic Community in creating a large melting-pot of diffusing cultures. This may in itself cause particular problems in treatment as alcohol use itself may be anathema to parents of young people who may have adopted a Western-style drinking culture. Problems may include disbelief and rejection of the person by the family, parents blaming each other for the problem and the problem drinker being kept a family secret. Family members, including the one with the drinking problem, may start to act dysfunctionally, spreading blame on each other which causes a rift in the once cohesive unit.

A further problem may emerge when alcohol use is entirely forbidden to protect other members of the family from suffering the same fate. This will eventually lead to those both with and without a drinking problem coming into conflict with parents and extended family.

Self-assessment question

What *are* the facts? Check your perceptions against those of the client and significant others.

Cultures are constantly evolving and changing due to globalisation. Someone raised in one culture may move to a new state or country and assimilate components of the new environment that were previously considered taboo or shameful but are accepted in their new home. Their original cultural heritage may either diminish or become extinct. Due to significant differences even between regions of the same state or country, people behave differently when dealing with issues around alcohol.

There are many barriers to communicating across cultures. The following are some of the main ones but the list is by no means exhaustive. The following barriers have been identified as important issues in assisting professionals who work with clients from other cultures:[5]

- *Language difference* doesn't just refer to the difference between being able to or not able to speak the dominant language. It refers also to dialect differences, the effect of jargon and or idioms and whether or not the individual is able to read and or write in their first, as well as their second, language.
- *Cultural difference* – Culture determines our expectations of how things will happen, what is considered polite or rude and what is 'understood' without saying a word. It relates not only to ethnicity but also to gender, class, education and environmental factors.
- *Non-verbal communication* – Gestures, expressions and body language can easily be misinterpreted. The most commonly cited example is the tendency in some cultures for people to avoid eye contact, as a sign of respect.
- *Stereotyping* – Belief about members of a group which is inadequately grounded, and at least partially inadequate because of overgeneralisation, but which the individual chooses not to change despite the facts.
- *Evaluating prejudice* – Judging someone's behaviour based on inadequate and usually stereotypical information.
- *Stress* is potentially present in all forms of communication, and is heightened by the presence of anxiety, pain, illness and other barriers to communication.
- *Organisational constraints* – Bureaucratic systems, no matter how honourable their missions, often make real communication difficult for both professionals and clients (e.g. complex 'legalese' forms).
- *The human factor* – Despite, or perhaps in addition to, a person's ethnicity there are individual human beings with a distinct personality which in itself may cause communication difficulties.
- *Resistance to change* – We live in the midst of change. In many individuals change is accompanied by feelings of confusion and fear of the unknown. In an attempt to regain the control they feel they have lost, individuals may resist the change and cling to structures and habits of their idealised past.

Self-assessment questions

1 How can we assist clients to fully tell their story?
2 What differences in body language have we noted amongst difference cultures?

Before we can work with the client we must have an understanding of, and sensitivity to, cultures other than our own. Treating all clients alike is unlikely to be effective. To work effectively with our clients we need to be aware of the differences and similarities between racial and ethnic groups. This cannot be learned alone, or in books or school, but through communication and hands-on experience with different groups. On the other hand we need to be alert to generalisations and ethnic stereotyping being created, and not allowing individual differences, particularly when dealing with alcohol and related issues.

Ethnic minority clients often need help to access, utilise and understand services available. It appears community-based and owned programmes are effective. Communities recognise the relationship between the person, their behaviour and the environment. They are also cost efficient, easily copied and can reach large numbers of people.[4]

Community rather than organisational ownership helps strengthen specific cultural elements in the communities, and may make them more attractive and user-friendly to those who would not normally use them, and those who would use nothing else.

In the past many different groups have not had access to culturally sensitive support for alcohol-related issues. Now with the advent of culturally sensitive, community-based programmes, there is more support, political power, authority, communication and direction in dealing with alcohol in our culturally diverse society.

One of the challenges is to find professionals who are skilled in both culturally sensitive issues and Western methods, so these could be combined and a specialist programme formulated and implemented by culturally trained persons.

Working with clients from cross-cultural backgrounds such as American Indians, Vietnamese, Australian indigenous Aborigines, Lebanese and Canadian Indians can present many potential problems. Language and cultural difference is one of the major ones, as may be age and gender; a person's dress or their ethnic background may be in conflict with the client's culture, for example Macedonians and Greeks, Jews and Palestinians. Much of this grows out of ethnocentrism, the belief that one's own group is superior, but may, however, spring from conflict in one's family of origin such as civil war, issues over sovereignty, displacement and other issues. It must be accepted that there may be occasions when cultural competency is not enough. Your culture may be rejected outright by the client. In these circumstances one should ensure that another staff member takes over.

It would be of great advantage to have workers who are culturally competent in order to bring together relevant areas of expertise in alcohol issues and cultural sensitivities, which would lead to community partnership, planning and implementation – the best of both worlds.

As professionals, we bring our own ethnocentrism with us in our work. The use of some strategies may have the opposite effect of that intended. For example, the recommendation that an American Indian client should attend a self-help group where the individual may be expected to expound on what alcohol has done to him or her and accept powerlessness over it, may have a negative effect on the person's self-esteem. The individual may treat the issue as a loss rather than a gain. However, the referral may be appropriate where the self-help group is a culturally based.

We may have a tolerant view of alcohol use but may deal with families where any use of alcohol is abhorrent. Our value may be that this is not a big issue, but the issue goes to the very cultural foundations of that family. Our values may be demonstrated where what we offer the client is based on our world view which stems from our own ethnocentrism. This means that the clients don't have what they need, the resources are applied inefficiently, and that benefits that may arise out of having an appropriate model spread via word of mouth through the community are lost.

It is not uncommon for clients to be unable or too terrified to verbally communicate their innermost feelings. Feelings are not only communicated verbally but through posture, eyes, expressions, gestures and much more. American Indians are culturally conditioned not to display public emotions and to avoid expressive gestures such as direct eye or physical contact in public. They are also compelled to fulfil the wishes of friends and relatives.[6] Learning how to see and be in touch with our clients is just as important as their spoken word.

However, our understanding of the spoken word needs to accept that cultural conversational styles are quite unique. Tannen[7] refers to linguists Ron and Susan Scollon, who found that:

> 'midwestern Americans, who may find themselves interrupted in conversations with Easterners, become aggressive interrupters when they talk to Athabaskan Indians, who expect much longer pauses. Many Americans find themselves interrupting when they talk to Scandinavians, but Swedes and Norwegians are perceived as interrupting by the longer-pausing Finns, who are themselves divided by regional differences with regard to the length of pauses and rate of speaking. As a result, Finns from certain parts of the country are stereotyped as fast-talking and pushy, and those from other parts of the

country are stereotyped as slow-talking and stupid, according to Finnish linguists, Jaakko Lehtonen and Kari Sajavarra.'

We must recognise the need to consider the culture of the person and frame questions accordingly. For example, to ask someone 'How much do you drink?' could be an insulting question and culturally inappropriate.

Self-assessment questions

1 Does your conversational style promote or hinder communication?
2 Is your format and process right for a particular client?
3 Do you need to change the process to facilitate effective cross-cultural communication?

What does alcohol use mean? In context, what is use for some is misuse for others. For example, when taking a history from a client and asking the amount of alcohol that they drink, they may use the term 'a normal amount' or 'I'm a social drinker'. This can have an entirely different meaning within each social grouping. In today's multicultural society there are cultures within cultures, within cultures, so that even within families let alone within countries one may find entirely different cultural expectations in relation to alcohol use.

Alcohol forms an important part of many rituals and indeed in some cultures would be seen as an integral part of celebration, and in others anathema. Among orthodox Jews, alcohol is used as a ritual beverage on sacral occasions, but it plays no role whatsoever in the daily calorie intake. In Italy, wine is mainly used as a food stuff. Alcohol is celebrated as part of the ritual of the Christian mass. Bottles of wine, never intended to be drunk, are auctioned for thousands of dollars. It can be a symbolism of sharing, birth, death and special events. It can be part of a country's economy. For some families it is the very livelihood on which the family is sustained – the growth of the produce.

Taboos and social norms are used to control alcohol use by cultures that fear it as an insidious drug:

> *'A Moroccan or Israeli man is labelled an incipient problem drinker if he averages more than two beers a week at anything other than formal social occasions, and a Sri Lankan woman seems abnormal if she drinks at all. In Ireland, Finland and elsewhere, drinking (at least in public) was a male prerogative until after World War II.'*[8]

However a different view:

> *'Among those who think at all about cross-cultural similarities and differences, it is widely assumed that men tend to monopolise access to alcohol, often forbidding women to drink. The reality is otherwise ... women have been drinking as long as men have throughout history, and they drink about as often as men in many cultures; in a few instances, they even seem to drink more, in spite of the fact that the physical impact of a given dose of alcohol is greater for women. In non-industrial societies, women usually have more easy access to alcohol beverages, in fact they often monopolise production and predominate in the distribution system.'*[9]

Looking at today's women, some would say there has been a marked increase in their consumption of alcohol, sometimes leading to major problems, and this may be due to the stress of juggling work both at and away from home. In other cultures, low rates of female alcohol use may be attributed to women having minimal if no free time to themselves.

Self-assessment question

Examine if any errors of language, perception, truth or logic are affecting your ability to assist a particular client.

Another important transcultural issue is that of alcohol use and violence. Five propositions on intoxication and aggression suggest:[10]

1 Alcohol-related behaviour is at least partly learned and is not the same in all cultures and communities; expectations about how intoxicated people will behave influence the way in which they do in fact behave.
2 Alcohol is widely used as an excuse for behaviour that may otherwise be unacceptable (the notion of time out).
3 The link between alcohol and violence is strongest in societies which manifest or endorse high levels of violent behaviour.
4 Those societies where alcohol is 'well integrated' into community life experience the fewest social problems (for example, violence) with alcohol.
5 Alcohol-related aggression is frequently associated with stress and or social or economic disadvantage.

It is important to remember that the above are only some factors, and are not without controversy. There is more support for some than others. However, propositions such as the above may help us understand alcohol-related violence as experienced by different communities in today's complex society.

Alcohol use has divided but has also united people in quite different ways, for example wine clubs and Alcoholics Anonymous.

If you take different points in time you can look at distinct differing influences, but now with globalisation, and with Europe becoming more of a community, there may be less cultural distinction and, as time goes on, fewer differences. This dilution of cultures was not seen a few generations ago. It has negative but also positive effects in dealing with alcohol use, and can cause intrafamiliar differences based on the old culture and the hybrid culture of migrant children.

The use of alcohol has often been subject to legislation in terms of age, so that the law has taken a view on what for many people is part of their culture. Many would not consider it abuse to give a child a watered-down glass of wine – but what if it is against the law? Thus, in some countries, the law may have intruded on culture.

Conclusion

Anyone working cross-culturally should have skills that help them to work with culturally diverse clientele. A commitment to cultural pluralism is shown by those who demonstrate a willingness both to accept change and to change themselves. As professionals, it is important to accept and understand our clients' cultural reality. Our relationship with our clients should not require either party to compromise their own beliefs and values.

If we wish to support our clients in dealing with alcohol issues within their communities, we need to be aware of the differing needs of these communities and the social diversity of the groups and different subgroups within it.

It is important we respect different cultural group decisions about what is a problem for their community and what is not. This can be difficult at times with our own agendas present. When communities decide there is a problem we should offer support, advice and resources as appropriate.

Knowledge of transcultural issues is the foundation on which we can build interpersonal and inter-group support and behaviours.

Taking cultural factors into account, which includes cultural diversity, respecting religious systems and rituals, understanding gender roles and family dynamics, appreciating the different political and legal systems which migrants may have experienced and putting aside our cultural stereotypes, enables us to facilitate access to the services we provide, to discover from clients the meaning they give to certain things, and to not make culturally based assumptions in advance.[5]

To develop your knowledge in this area, see 'To learn more', p. 259.

Self-assessment questions

1 Are you comfortable with your own cultural identity?
2 Is your appearance culturally appropriate to work with your client? (This would mean not appropriating dress and customs of cultures we may work with but are not a part of.)
3 Is there a status of elder within the culture you are working with? (If so, how can you best use that person? Their input may validate the services on offer and their acceptance may be needed in order to assist communities in developing their own services.)
4 Has your relationship with a particular client been one that has fostered a positive self-image?
5 List ways in which your service can be improved to work with culturally diverse clients.
6 List services which you have not used before but know would be useful in providing culturally sensitive services to clients.
7 In developing further programmes, list some of the critical elements in planning appropriate cultural services.

CHAPTER 11

The workplace, employer and employee

*Paul M Roman, J Aaron Johnson
and Terry C Blum*

Acknowledgement

The authors gratefully acknowledge the support of Grant R01-AA-10130 from the National Institute on Alcohol Abuse and Alcoholism during the preparation of this manuscript.

Pre-reading exercise

This exercise should take no more than 20 minutes. When you have read the chapter, repeat the exercise to see if your understanding is the same or has increased.

Research has shown that many factors affect drinking. Most of the emphases are upon genetic, familial and social learning factors. We know, however, that increasing proportions of the world's adults spend a major part of their waking hours at work. What aspects of workplaces might influence an employee to increase or decrease alcohol consumption?

Introduction

The alcohol and workplace relationship can be approached from two broad perspectives. First, there is a wealth of research examining alcohol use as a dependent variable. Certain occupations, job characteristics or organisational structures may increase alcohol consumption or problem drinking among individuals employed in those settings. Second, there is an extensive literature which treats alcohol use as a causal variable, looking at how alcohol use and abuse shapes the organisational structure of the workplace through generating programmes to address the impacts of problem drinking. Here we address only the impact of work and the workplace on alcohol use, suggesting additional reading at the end of the chapter references covering both substantive areas.

Historical background

Alcohol has long been an accompaniment of work, and in this role has not always been problematic. The global community that has emerged over recent decades has blunted the cross-cultural differences in drinking patterns and in the associations between work and drinking. Generally, the alcohol and work linkage is forbidden or strongly discouraged, but the use of alcohol in conjunction with work is not yet unknown around the world.

The key to understanding the changes in this linkage is technology involving machines and symbol manipulation. It is not only machines that reduced the tolerance for work-related drinking, but also the kinds of work organisations that were the consequences of machine technology. Without the need to 'rest', without concerns about the needs of smaller machines that are dependent on larger machines for sustenance, and without interest in leisure or recreation, machines allow for the continuous operation. This feature led to new concepts of time associated with work, distinguishing between work time and non-work time, establishing 'shifts' for round-the-clock work periods, and eventually yielding for many non-work days or weeks known as vacations.

Machines can keep up a pace of activity that does not parallel human capability. While there are some exceptions (such as computer programs that will automatically correct minor spelling errors while typing proceeds), most machine activity does not detect or react to boredom or inattention among human operators. While there are effective safety devices, many machines do not instantly stop operation when there is evidence of peril to human life or limb. The automobile is a prime example of such an unresponsive, intolerant and therefore menacing machine.

We do not need to belabour these examples to make it clear that when work becomes organised around machine activity, the tolerance for impairment of human operators by psychoactive substance use disappears. Workers whose cognitive and motor processes are affected by alcohol and other drugs put themselves at menace when interacting with machines. From an efficiency perspective, such impaired operators also risk errors in operating the machine or damage to it through faulty judgement. Finally, when we look at the importance of time in the contemporary organisation of work, it is clear that the hung-over worker or the worker who drinks during the workday is likely going to be a problematic absentee or incompetent, creating concerns not only for supervisors but also for co-workers who are 'pulling their own weight'.

For most in industrial societies at the close of the millennium, it is difficult to imagine work environments where drinking was acceptable and even encouraged.[1] Such an understanding requires that we dismiss from our minds the large workplaces of the contemporary scene, the generally impersonal relations between employers and employees, and the ideas of time-clocks, shifts and even workdays.

Pre-machine techniques in agriculture, for example, required extensive human labour, but presented relatively few risks to workers. Agricultural workers were nearly always dependent upon harvests for their direct livelihood, and when crops failed, starvation loomed. Time was significant as represented by seasons and weather, with some times of the year and some weather conditions calling for work from dawn to dusk or even longer, while other seasons and weather conditions precluded work altogether. It should be evident that drinking in conjunction with work during this pre-industrial period was not problematic as compared to machine technologies operating in today's large work organisations.

In the pre-machine era, there were many activities that were not agricultural, but these craft and professional activities also involved very simple technologies, generally non-threatening to human well-being. The pace of work was determined by the demand for products, and without large-scale marketing and distribution systems, demand stayed close to sustenance levels. This allowed workers and their helpers to have a high degree of control over how and when work was done.

Thus, the relation between alcohol and work has been dramatically altered by technology, and the impact of technology on the organisation of work. These two macro-level forces have in turn affected and been affected by cultural norms about appropriate and inappropriate drinking behaviour. Whereas the authors of the American Constitution and the intellectuals of 17th and 18th-century London kept their thoughts well lubricated with alcohol throughout the workday, the world of today would find such behaviour unacceptable and licentious.

There are potentially important lessons in these historical changes. As we look about us at employed people whose behaviour involves excessive drinking off the job, or even drinking on the job, we can ask the extent to which their immediate work environments are similar or dissimilar to the pre-machine work epoch. Such considerations are also important in countries where economic development is occurring rapidly, with introduction of widespread machine technology. In some instances, wages are providing ready access to alcohol within cultures where norms have restricted drinking generally or compartmentalised drinking to ritual occasions. In these settings alcohol distributors are both creating and responding to market demands, suggesting the eventual emergence of significant social problems.[2]

The impact of the workplace on alcohol use

Studies of the epidemiology of alcohol problems and the workplace date back more than 150 years.[3] Research in this area has revolved around four major perspectives or hypotheses: cultural, social control or self-selection, alienation and work stress.[4] Proponents of the cultural perspective assert that subcultures develop within certain industries and or worksites. These subcultures form group norms about what constitutes normal drinking. The social control or self-selection perspective holds that individuals prone to heavy drinking select occupations that facilitate their drinking habits and their desire to continue a pattern of heavy drinking. This leads that person to select an occupation with limited supervision, low visibility of job performance or ready access to alcohol (e.g. bartending). Both the proponents of the alienation and work stress perspectives believe that some occupational and job characteristics have a significant impact on an employee's alcohol consumption. Drawing from the work of Marx and other critical theorists, researchers adopting the alienation perspective argue that work roles lacking creativity, variety and independent judgement create in workers a sense of dissatisfaction and powerlessness that they learn to relieve through drinking.[5] By contrast, researchers adopting the work stress perspective do not assume that work is central to one's identity. They do believe that a variety of workplace stressors (monotony, complexity, control of tasks, etc.) may directly or indirectly impact alcohol consumption.

Unfortunately, the absence of longitudinal research in this field has made it difficult to verify any single perspective. For example, researchers have identified a number of occupations characterised by high levels of alcohol consumption and a high prevalence of alcohol problems.[6,7] Because of the absence of longitudinal data, these researchers have been unable to establish whether these occupations are subcultures which 'socialise' employees into their established drinking norms (cultural perspective) or if the employee has selected the occupation because it offers the opportunity for high levels of alcohol consumption with little chance of detection (social control perspective).

Perhaps the foremost proponents of the cultural perspective are Ames and her associates.[7-9] They argue that drinking subcultures are developed and maintained in work-related environments and serve both symbolic and actual functions in the work organisation.[7] Within these subcultures, drinking becomes normative behaviour and contributes to group solidarity and job identity. A classic example of this phenomenon is described by Sonnenstuhl and Trice[10] in their study of the New York City tunnel and construction workers ('sandhogs'). For the sandhogs, the group's solidarity revolved around heavy drinking. Sonnenstuhl and Trice,[10] along with other studies, find that workers whose social support networks centre around co-workers drink more heavily and report more drinking-related problems than workers whose primary reference group is not work-based. However, the impact of drinking norms is not unidirectional, as Sonnenstuhl[11] later described the emergence of a sobriety subculture among sandhogs who had affiliated with Alcoholics Anonymous (AA).

Howland et al.[12] also report evidence of workplace drinking subcultures. Collecting data from 114 worksites representing seven corporations, they find significant differences in reported alcohol consumption across the worksites. Given the diversity of their sample (as contrasted to the research of Ames et al. in a single corporation), their findings suggest that drinking subcultures may emerge at separate worksites even within the same corporation.

Delaney and Ames[9] argue that one way of preventing the development of these drinking subcultures is through the implementation of work teams. In their study of perceived workplace drinking norms they find that employees involved in work teams and with positive team attitudes report less perceived permissiveness of workplace drinking. Employees who are involved in their teams, feel their input is valued and believe their teams are effective see their team members and supervisors as intolerant of on-the-job alcohol use.[9]

For workers with pre-existing alcohol problems, the implementation of work teams may have the opposite effect. For example, Roman et al.[13] find evidence to suggest co-workers and supervisors can serve as 'enablers' for employees whose performance has been affected by problem drinking. 'Enabling' describes the process whereby social networks (family, co-workers, etc.) assist the problem drinker in maintaining the appearance of normal functioning. Enabling thus delays the identification of, and intervention in, problem drinking behaviour. In the case of the workplace, enabling is characterised by co-workers and supervisors 'covering' for the problem drinker's absences and or decline in productivity. Using longitudinal data from the 1973 and 1977 Quality of Employment Survey, Roman et al.[13] find problem drinkers more likely to report a perception of increased workgroup assistance behaviour. While the data were limited, these findings point to the possibility of enabling being variable across different workgroup cultures.

As mentioned earlier, the lack of longitudinal research makes it difficult to test the social control perspective. While Parker and Harford[5] identify a number of occupations with unusually high average daily consumption levels and or a high prevalence of alcohol dependence (bartenders, food service workers, fishers, forestry workers, farmers, etc.), it is unclear whether fellow employees in these occupations convert the individual to their drinking norms or whether these occupations are purposefully selected by the problem drinker because of their 'low visibility'. Clearly some of these occupations (fishers, forestry workers, farmers, etc.) are such that the employee could easily conceal alcohol use or alcohol-related problems. Manello and Seaman[14] found lack of supervision to be a prominent factor in drinking among railroad workers. Ames and Janes[15] corroborate Manello and Seaman's findings in a study of automobile workers. However, both these studies were qualitative studies of blue-collar occupations. Qualitative studies are unable to identify other possible independent variables such as level of extrinsic rewards, pace of work, co-worker relations, etc. Other research has found that these latter characteristics affect individual patterns of alcohol consumption.[16–19]

One glaring problem with the social control perspective is that in order to accept the perspective, the researcher must make two assumptions. First, the researcher must assume that, prior to employment, the prospective employee is aware of the 'permissive' characteristics of the occupation. Second, the researcher must assume that, even if aware of these characteristics, the prospective employee is able to obtain his/her desired occupation. Both these assumptions are tenuous at best.

Perhaps the most promising avenue of research on the impact of the workplace on alcohol use has been the alienation and work stress perspective. As mentioned earlier, these two perspectives are very similar and will therefore be addressed simultaneously. Because of the large proportion of an individual's life devoted to one's occupation, researchers have long argued that work will play a significant role in shaping the individual's overall life quality. An occupation viewed as rewarding by the employee (both substantively and monetarily) is likely to have a positive impact on the overall mental health of the individual. Conversely, a job characterised by a high level of job stress, 'burnout' and poor wages may impact the individual's mental and or physical health in a negative way.

Numerous studies have examined the impact of work and the workplace on employees' mental health and, more specifically, employee drinking patterns.[4,18–25] Contemporary research centres around the belief that individuals working in non-rewarding occupations will attempt to relieve their dissatisfaction by increasing their consumption of alcohol. The consumption of alcohol off-the-job provides the worker with a mechanism for escaping, forgetting or redefining the effects of non-rewarding on-the-job experiences.[18]

Using data from a nationally representative sample of employed men, Martin *et al.*[18] find that one of the most important predictors of frequency and quantity of alcohol consumption is escapist drinking (drinking to forget about the job, forget about problems on the job, to relax, etc.). Furthermore, two job characteristics have significant effects on reported escapist reasons for drinking. Respondents are more likely to cite escapist reasons for drinking under conditions of high job pressure, and less likely to cite these reasons when levels of extrinsic rewards (good pay, good benefits, good job security) are high.[18] Martin *et al.* [19] extend their earlier research by identifying buffers to problem drinking. While job-escape drinking continues to be a concern, this more recent article finds that supportive co-workers reduce the likelihood of being classified as a problem drinker.[19] Consistent with earlier research,[10] Martin *et al.* [19] find that frequency of drinking when socialising with co-workers away from work positively influences problem drinking.

While Martin and his associates find a marginal but significant relationship between job stress, escape drinking and problem drinking, other research does not support these findings. Cooper *et al.* [26] find little support for the belief that work stress promotes problematic alcohol use. In a test of social learning theory, they argue that the 'real-world impact of work stressors on alcohol-related outcomes is likely to be small [p. 270]'.[26]

While Martin *et al.* [19] utilise data from a nationally representative sample of full-time employees, most research in this area has been based on non-representative samples in single industries. Influenced by Marx's argument that alienation should be prominent among the proletariat employed in intrinsically non-rewarding jobs, most of these researchers have focused exclusively on blue-collar occupations. However, Richman and her colleagues[27,28] argue that stress and alienation are not exclusive to low-status workers. Using longitudinal data collected from medical school students from the time they entered medical school through their first year as interns, Richman *et al.* [28] find that abusive experiences such as sexual harassment, discriminatory treatment and psychological humiliations predict various drinking outcomes (problem drinking, escape drinking, frequency drinking, quantity drinking) in both male and female medical students. What is important about Richman's work is its experiential focus rather than reliance on reports of job characteristics or attitudinal measures. Whereas earlier studies of blue-collar workers hypothesised that high workload demands increase employee alcohol consumption, Richman[27] finds that among medical students heavy workloads serve to constrain alcohol use rather than promote it.

The alcohol and work relationship among special populations

The effect of employment on female drinking patterns

As the percentage of women employed outside the home has risen over the past several decades, there has been an increased concern over the effects that employment has had on women, particularly those employed in occupations that have traditionally been male-dominated. One concern is that, while problem drinking among women has traditionally been low compared to their male counterparts, increased participation in the workforce may result in a convergence of the male : female problem-drinking ratio. The potential for such a convergence is particularly troubling given the apparent dangers associated with alcohol use by expectant mothers.

Studies show that the drinking patterns of employed women are different from those of women not employed outside the home.[29-31] Employed women are less likely to be abstinent, and report greater frequency and quantity of alcohol consumption.[32] However, employed men continue to consume more alcohol and have more alcohol-related problems than their employed female counterparts. Is this increased consumption a result of increased stress or merely a function of employed women's increased access to alcohol? Because working women frequently perform a number of other roles (mother, housewife, spouse, etc.), a number of studies have hypothesised that increased drinking may result from having too many roles (role overload) or from having roles that place competing demands on the person (role conflict).[30,32,33] Most findings indicate that neither role overload nor role conflict are significant predictors of employed women's increased alcohol consumption.[29,30,32] In fact, multiple roles may benefit, rather than threaten, women's health. Richman's[27,28] work cited earlier indicates that heavier demands on people may actually preclude occasions for drinking.

While women in female-dominated jobs report lower levels of alcohol use than those employed in male-dominated jobs, Shore[32] attributes this to perceived social disapproval of women's drinking and traditional feminine values in female-dominated jobs. Among women in male-dominated jobs, more frequent opportunities to drink and traditional masculine values predominate.[32] Such differences imply that increased alcohol consumption among employed women may be due to increased opportunity to drink and increased accessibility to drink, rather than role conflict and or role overload.

Alcohol use among recent workforce entrants

Of particular interest, but less widely studied, are the consumption patterns of recent workforce entrants. Given the centrality of the work ethic in Western society, these cultures tend to encourage youthful employment and behaviours that may be seen as precursors for adult careers. However, among teens, employment is strongly correlated with alcohol use and abuse.[34–36] Steinberg and colleagues[34] find that previously unemployed teenagers who were employed at the one-year follow-up were using alcohol and drugs significantly more often than their counterparts who had remained unemployed. Furthermore, as the number of work hours increases, teenagers report higher rates of alcohol and drug use.[35] Using data from the National Household Survey on Drug Abuse (NHSDA), Roman and Johnson[36] find that employed male and female teenagers are significantly more likely than their non-employed peers to be classified as heavy or moderate drinkers while non-employed teenagers are more likely to report being abstainers.

Taking these findings one step further, employed teenagers who subsequently experience the early onset of drinking problems may be less likely to continue their education beyond high school. This implication seems to be supported by the research on young adults conducted by both Sanford and colleagues[37] and Mullahy and Sindelar.[38,39] Sanford *et al.*[37] find that young people engaged in heavy substance use are significantly less likely to be in school. Mullahy and Sindelar[38,39] find that early onset of alcohol problems is correlated with lower levels of education. Furthermore, as the findings of Sanford *et al.*[37] appear to support, teenagers who experience an early onset of drinking problems may find themselves unemployed as young adults if they have been unable to bring their drinking under control. Confirmation of these implications requires longitudinal data following both employed and unemployed teenagers for at least a decade, and such data do not yet exist.

These findings appear to contradict the popular conception that teen employment outside the home instills discipline and responsibility. Instead, these findings suggest that employed teenagers are more highly involved in alcohol use than their non-employed peers and that such involvement seems to increase as work hours increase. Steinberg and Dornbusch[35] offer three possible explanations for this discrepancy: (1) workers have more discretionary income to use for purchasing alcohol, (2) workers experience more stress than non-workers and consequently use alcohol as a means of coping with this additional stress, and (3) workers encounter older adolescents and young adults in the workplace who expose them to drinking activities. Note that the second and third reasons correspond to the work stress and cultural perspectives, respectively.

Unfortunately, the majority of the studies in this area, including the research conducted by Mullahy and Sindelar,[38,39] have relied on cross-sectional data and, as such, provide a limited picture of the alcohol and work relationship. Consequently, it is difficult to specify a causal direction for the alcohol and work relationship among teenagers and young adults. It seems logical, however, that the relationship could be bidirectional. Based on any of the reasons suggested by Steinberg and Dornbusch,[35] teen employment could lead to increases in alcohol consumption. In turn, those teens and young adults who engage in heavy alcohol use or abuse may be less likely to either continue in school or obtain a white-collar job.

As a result, some of these young problem drinkers may become locked into a lifelong existence in the lower class, a hypothesis supported by Vaillant's[40] longitudinal research. His data indicate that although most lower class boys could improve their socio-economic status as adults, those boys with low intelligence, psychiatric disorders, alcohol dependence or a combination of such factors are found in the lower class as adults, regardless of their original socio-economic background.

The absence of work: the effect of retirement on elderly alcohol consumption

In considering the effects of alcohol use and abuse among older adults, several inherent factors contribute to an overall decrease in alcohol consumption among this population. First, adults age 60 or older are unlikely to be heavy drinkers, simply because the heaviest drinkers tend to succumb at an earlier age to physical complications, accidents or other injuries related to excessive alcohol consumption.[41,42] Also, the ageing process results in decreased physical tolerance for alcohol's effects during and after drinking episodes, leading to reduced consumption both on a voluntary basis and from advice from significant others.

Much speculation but sparse facts exist regarding the effects of occupational retirement on alcohol consumption. For many people, retirement may be a particularly stressful period in which they experience a loss of status, boredom, depression, loss of self-esteem or general discordance as to what their roles are as members of society.[43] Researchers conjecture that retirees turn to alcohol to help them cope with this stress.[43,44] In addition, researchers speculate that older men may be more at risk for such stress-related alcohol abuse than older women, because men, particularly the current generation of retirees, tend to be more highly integrated into the labour force and are more likely to hold high-status managerial jobs. At retirement, this status loss may be especially difficult for men to accept.

In addition to increased stress, the retiree is afforded more leisure time in which to consume alcohol. With few role constraints or social obligations, the retiree may consume alcohol with greatly reduced risks of adverse social consequences.[43] Because men report higher levels of alcohol consumption than women throughout life,[45] leisure-related alcohol consumption associated with retirement also may occur more frequently among men than women.

In the Normative Aging Study, Ekerdt *et al.*[43] attempt to address the effects of retirement on alcohol consumption systematically by assessing pre- and post-retirement change in male retirees' drinking behaviours. The group of retirees was then compared with a similar group of age peers who continued to work. Although the study data are based on a small sample size and a single geographical location, Ekerdt *et al.*[43] find that retirement is not associated with a change in average alcohol consumption. They did find, however, that retirees show greater variability over time in consumption levels: a number of retirees reported heavy drinking patterns, whereas others reported the cessation of heavy drinking and its related problems. Finally, retirees are more likely than their employed age peers to report the onset of periodic heavier drinking and drinking problems.[43]

In contrast, other researchers suggest that a significant decrease occurs in the level of alcohol consumption as people approach retirement age.[46,47] This decline may be attributed to a number of factors. Retirement may eliminate the job stress which, as previously discussed, is correlated with heavy drinking; retirement may also remove people from workplace drinking subcultures, such as those discussed in the work of Ames and her colleagues.[7-9] After leaving such an environment, retirees may reduce their alcohol consumption levels substantially. For many older adults, another possible contributor to the decline in alcohol consumption is reduced income during retirement, which financially may limit their access to alcoholic beverages.

Barnes[46] strongly argues that retirement is not related to an increase in heavy drinking. She finds that adults over age 60 who are still employed are twice as likely to be heavy drinkers as those who are unemployed or retired. Roman and Johnson[36] corroborate Barnes's[46] findings. Using data from a nationally representative sample, they find that employed males and females over age 60 are significantly more likely than their unemployed peers to be classified as heavy or moderate drinkers. Complementing these results is the research of Mullahy and Sindelar,[39] who observe that alcohol abusers tend to remain in the labour force longer than non-alcoholics. The researchers reason that workers without alcohol problems are able to accrue greater wealth and larger pensions than alcoholics and therefore may retire, whereas the person with alcohol-related problems must continue to work.

In summary, stress and additional leisure time associated with retirement may adversely affect some older people by increasing their alcohol consumption to an abusive level, but the extent of such a pattern may not be large. Only Ekerdt *et al.*[43] find that retirees are likely to experience the onset of periodic heavy drinking. Gurnack and Hoffman[48] attribute abusive drinking among retirees to a history of alcohol abuse, not to age-related stress. Barnes[46] as well as Roman and Johnson[36] show that employed older adults, rather than retirees, are more likely to report high levels of alcohol consumption.

Most of the current literature on elderly alcohol consumption suffers from the same basic limitations as the more general literature on the alcohol and work relationship. First, findings are tenuous because data are cross-sectional and therefore unable to establish causality. Second, most data are limited to a single industry or geographical location, making generalisations impossible. These limitations must be resolved before findings on the relationship between retirement and alcohol-related problems among the older adult population can be considered conclusive.

Conclusion

The linkage between alcohol and work is significant but understudied. There are a number of exciting hypotheses, but few opportunities to test these ideas in longitudinal designs. The focus of research on the chronic drinker and on high-risk populations draws attention away from the very important social fact that most drinkers work and are impacted by work-related forces on almost a daily basis. Further, work is dynamic, for people have careers wherein conditions of work change about them as the dynamics of adult development generate parallel changes.

In this chapter we have highlighted aspects of the historical relationship between work and alcohol, the possible impacts of work on drinking and the characteristics of the work and alcohol relationship among employed women, young workers and retirees. Clearly, the extant literature raises more questions than it answers, but there can be no doubt that the questions raised are exciting and important.

To develop your knowledge in this area, see 'To learn more', p. 262.

Self-assessment questions

1 Why don't we design machine technology to be more 'friendly' to persons consuming alcohol?
2 How would drinking be rewarding to persons who are alienated from their jobs?

3 Thinking about the life cycle, what age-level of worker is going to be the most vulnerable to norms about drinking in the workplace?
4 Under what conditions would 'too much work' possibly cause one to drink and under what conditions would it prevent people from drinking?
5 What types of retirees would you expect to be at the greatest risk for developing drinking problems?

PART TWO

Responses to the related problems

CHAPTER 12

Prevention, intervention, education and health promotion

Hazel E Watson

Pre-reading exercise

Before reading this chapter, take time to answer the following questions. When you have read the chapter, repeat the exercise to see if your understanding has improved. This exercise should take no more than 15 minutes.

1 What is meant by the term 'problem drinking'?
2 What picture does this term conjure up in your mind?
3 What is meant by the term 'sensible drinking'?
4 At what age do you think people should be made aware of sensible drinking limits, and whose responsibility is this?

Introduction

In previous chapters of this book, the effects of alcohol consumption on physical, psychological and social well-being have been described. In this chapter, issues which relate to the prevention of problem drinking and the promotion of sensible drinking will be discussed.

The prevalence of alcohol-related health problems is increasing in both the developed and developing world and now constitutes a major cause of morbidity and mortality.[1-3] Problem drinkers themselves experience the adverse effects of excessive drinking. However, just as passive smoking by non-smokers causes health problems, problem drinkers also cause problems to others in society, such as the families, friends and colleagues of those who drink excessively. The costs to individuals, families and societies are considerable.[4,5]

Because people with alcohol-related problems do not often seek treatment until their problems are compounded by advanced physical, psychological and or social complications,[6-8] treatment is often unsuccessful and costly in terms of health service and voluntary organisation resources.[2,9] It is therefore appropriate for treatment approaches to alcohol problems to adopt strategies which encompass preventative measures and the early detection and interventions for problem drinking. In the *Alma Ata Declaration of Health for All by the Year 2000*, the World Health Organization raised the profile globally of such approaches to health problems which are associated with lifestyle factors, including excessive alcohol consumption.[10]

At a general population level, individuals who are habitual heavy drinkers and have multiple health and social alcohol-related problems represent a relatively small proportion of those who consume alcohol. In contrast, the majority of alcohol-related disabilities are caused by moderate drinkers.[11] It has been calculated that an average reduction in alcohol consumption by all drinkers of 10% would result in a 25% reduction in problem drinking.[12] This surely, then, justifies a wider approach to health promotion, prevention and treatment than has previously been offered.

It is important to acknowledge that alcohol has been used in many societies since early civilisation. Its use has become inextricably interwoven into the fabric of the cultures of many nations. Although there are notable exceptions, alcohol has symbolic significance in many religious festivals and has long-standing associations with the national traditions and ceremonies of many countries. The majority of people who drink alcohol do so in moderation and their drinking is an enjoyable and low-risk activity which contributes positively to social recreation. As such, it is appropriate to maintain a balanced perspective on health promotion, with advice focusing on sensible drinking and harm reduction.

Sensible drinking

It has been argued that there is no such thing as safe drinking, since all drinking carries some risk to health and safety. For example, it is never advisable to drink before or during work since even small amounts of alcohol consumed can affect a person's judgement. In the UK the Health Education Authority has published guidelines which indicate the relative risk to health which is associated with different levels of alcohol consumption. These are shown in Box 12.1. These levels were adopted from information in the reports of the Royal College of Physicians and the Royal College of General Practitioners, and have subsequently been endorsed by the British Medical Association.[13-15]

In the UK, one standard drink of alcohol contains 8 grams of ethanol (*see also* Chapter 2) and is equivalent to the following measures:

- half a pint of lager or light beer (3.5% alcohol content by volume)
- 25 ml of spirits
- 50 ml fortified wines (e.g. sherry, Martini)
- 125 ml table wine.

The authors of the Royal College reports recognise that there is a continuum for increasing risk associated with increasing consumption. They also emphasised the point that the limits of 21 standard drinks per week for men and 14 standard drinks per week for women are general guidelines only and do not take into account individual variations. There is also a danger that describing any level of consumption as 'sensible' may lead to people interpreting it as the level up to which drinking is problem-free. It is possible that such an interpretation may cause light drinkers to increase their level of consumption. In addition, young people as a group tend to be attracted to risk-taking and may be encouraged to drink to excess by the fact that the guidelines exist. However, on balance, despite these reservations, there are undoubted benefits in having such guidelines. They provide a focus for health education and can be used as a yardstick by which people can make decisions about how much they can drink without, in the majority of cases, adverse consequences to health.

Since the weekly limits were advocated there has been a recognition of the considerable risk to health which arises from 'binge' drinking, i.e. drinking the weekly limit or more in one drinking session.[16,17] Drinking relatively large amounts of alcohol, irrespective of whether this is a frequent occurrence, can lead to road traffic accidents, domestic violence and unruly and aggressive behaviour, all of which may incur personal injury, damage to property, or breach of the peace and involvement in criminal procedures. Consequently a daily, rather than weekly, limit is now recommended. The British Medical Association's sensible-drinking message is shown in Box 12.2.

Box 12.1 Health risk and levels of alcohol consumption

Risk	Men	Women
High	50 standard drinks per week or more	35 standard drinks per week or more
Moderate	21–49 standard drinks per week	14–34 standard drinks per week
Low	Less than 21 standard drinks per week	Less than 14 standard drinks per week

---

Box 12.2 British Medical Association's sensible-drinking message (Reproduced with kind permission of the British Medical Association.)

- Your risk of developing alcohol-related disease is low if you drink no more than:
  - women: 2 standard drinks per day (e.g. 2 small glasses of wine, 1 pint of ordinary strength beer, lager or cider, 2 single measures of spirits)
  - men: 3 standard drinks per day (e.g. 3 small glasses of wine, 1.5 pint of ordinary strength beer, lager or cider, 3 single measures of spirits).
- If you drink more than these amounts, you progressively increase the risk of harm to your health.
- Drinking within low-risk amounts (as above) may reduce the risk of heart disease.
- Drinking that causes drunkenness is dangerous to yourself, your family and society.
- Drinking and driving is dangerous and driving under the influence of alcohol is a criminal offence.
- Drinking before and during work is dangerous in some jobs and impairs judgement and effectiveness in all.

Prevention

Health promotion seeks to enhance positive health, while at the same time preventing ill health.[18] Health promotion activities encompass a wide range of activities which aim to maximise the health, well-being and quality of life of individuals and communities.[19] Armstrong and Robins maintain that since alcohol is part of our culture and society, society has a responsibility for those who suffer from its adverse effects.[20] It is therefore suggested that governments have a responsibility to support measures which prevent problem drinking. Such measures may include legal controls, resourcing national and local health promotion initiatives, and the provision of appropriate healthcare facilities.

Legal controls

Pricing strategies
Fiscal measures which governments impose include the taxation of alcoholic beverages. Studies conducted in the USA and the UK show that

increasing the cost of alcohol leads to a lower incidence of problems associated with drinking.[21] There is little evidence, however, that price rises cause heavy drinkers to cut down their consumption. Nonetheless, since taxes, which constitute revenue to governments, contribute a major proportion of the price of alcohol, rises in tax have the potential to reduce overall harm associated with alcohol consumption.

Purchasing restrictions

The age at which it is legal to buy alcohol is a further means by which governments can exert control over drinking. This varies from country to country. In most states of the USA this has recently been increased to 21 years, and there is evidence to suggest that this has reduced the number of alcohol-related deaths.[22] However, there is also concern that such restrictions lead to experimentation and excessive consumption by some adolescents. There is evidence of a dramatic rise in alcohol-related injuries attending the accident and emergency department of a children's hospital.[23]

Legal restrictions which impinge on alcohol consumption include the licensing of premises from which alcohol can be purchased, and also the imposition of limits on the length of time during which alcohol can be bought. Prohibition in the USA in the 1920s did indeed result in a reduction of the per capita rate of consumption as recorded by official statistics.[24] However, such data do not take cognisance of illegal production and consumption which may have been occurring at the time. Similar criticisms have been levelled at the effectiveness of the somewhat stringent restrictions on the availability of alcohol in some Scandinavian countries.[25] In Scotland, the law which controls the sale of alcohol was changed in 1976 with the effect that the hours during which alcohol could be purchased were extended. Although it is difficult to extrapolate the direct effects of such actions, there is no evidence of significant changes in alcohol consumption or alcohol-related harm occurring as a consequence of the change in the licensing laws.[26]

Standard drink labelling

In recent years there has been a move towards expressing the alcoholic content of different beverages as 'standard drinks' (*see also* Chapter 2), particularly when giving health education advice regarding sensible drinking. Governments throughout the Western world have been pressurised to pass legislation making it compulsory for labels to indicate the alcohol content of the product in 'standard drinks'. This has been achieved with little success to date, although some manufacturers have undertaken to do so of their own accord.

Unfortunately there is, as yet, no international agreement regarding the notional 'standard drink' (*see also* Chapter 2). For example, as indicated earlier in this chapter, the UK standard drink contains 8 grams of alcohol, whereas in Australia and New Zealand the standard drink refers to 10 grams. In Canada and the USA it is 13.6 and 14 grams respectively.[27] A more precise form of measurement would provide a useful base for health education purposes, and also with regard to the training needs of healthcare professionals and other interested parties. In addition, without true standardisation, it is difficult to compare the results of research studies which use different definitions of the standard drink of alcohol, making cross-cultural generalisations almost impossible (*see also* Chapter 2).

Health warning labelling
In many countries, such as the USA, Mexico and India, the labels of alcohol products carry health warnings. Since the majority of people who consume alcohol also purchase it, advocates of this strategy maintain that the health education message can reach the target audience for which it is intended. Furthermore, the wording of the message can be used to direct the reader to particular adverse effects of drinking and can therefore act as a specific health education intervention. It has been suggested that individuals who are not problem drinkers are most likely to heed the warnings.[28] In Britain, among other countries, there has been resistance to a legal requirement for such a measure, despite a vocal lobby.

National and local initiatives

By the age of eight years most children in the UK understand that alcohol is a special sort of beverage.[29] Consequently those concerned with promoting sensible drinking have argued that alcohol education should begin within the first few years of school. Nurses, and others who provide health and social care, should be involved in schools and other venues with children and parents, both individually and in local groups, to discuss the subject and to provide appropriate literature with the aim of promoting attitudes which are commensurate with sensible drinking.

Health education authorities in the UK are government-funded bodies which develop and provide health education materials, and also plan and organise national campaigns and promotional activities which can be taken up locally by healthcare activists to good effect.

The role of occupational health professionals has also developed in recent years, and the workplace is now an arena for the implementation of health-promoting activities. Given the adverse effects of excessive alcohol consumption on safety and effectiveness at work, there are strong ethical, and also economic, reasons for employers to support such measures.

Health screening clinics, which are offered in both primary, occupational and acute care settings, also offer opportunities for health promotion, as well as for the identification of those individuals whose level of alcohol consumption is a matter of concern.

Identifying problem drinkers

A number of studies have advocated the benefits of minimal, or brief, interventions which can be given in both primary care and general hospital settings by generalist practitioners, rather than those who have specialist skills in treating habitual or dependent drinkers.[30–34] Doctors, nurses and other members of the multidisciplinary team, working as they do in diverse healthcare settings, have opportunities to identify potential problem drinkers and provide appropriate advice[35,36] (*see also* Chapters 17 and 18).

In order to provide appropriate information for potential problem drinkers it is important to identify those whose level of consumption renders them at risk of developing alcohol-related problems. It has been suggested that health professionals should be alert to individuals who present with early indicators of problem drinking, such as gastrointestinal symptoms, recurrent accidents, anxiety, insomnia, sexual problems and family and work problems.[37] Patients who present with such problems should be assessed carefully. On the other hand, Murray[38] has advocated screening of all patients in primary healthcare and hospital settings to detect potential problem drinkers.[38]

Asking people how much alcohol they drink is the easiest way of determining risk. There is a general impression that people are reluctant to give a true account of how much they drink, and either evade the issue or provide unreliable information. However, there is good evidence to suggest that this is not the case and that the information which most people give is sufficiently truthful.[39,40]

Key point: Questions about alcohol consumption should be asked in a sensitive but matter-of-fact way when other lifestyle factors, such as diet, exercise and smoking, are asked as part of routine procedures on admission to hospital or when attending clinics at health centres or GP practices.[41]

When assessing alcohol consumption it is appropriate to note not only how much alcohol an individual consumes, but also the pattern of consumption. It is important to know this because it influences the nature of the advice which should be given. Binge drinkers, whose drinking is concentrated on one or two days per week, are likely to experience different problems from those who drink as much, but in smaller amounts on a more regular basis. For this reason, quantity and frequency measures, which are calculated by multiplying the average amount of alcohol consumed by the number of drinking days per week, are not advised.

Descriptive statements such as 'social' or 'heavy' drinker are not helpful as they are subjective and open to interpretation in different ways by different people. On the other hand, the use of an accepted system which measures consumption in 'standard drinks' of alcohol has the advantage of providing an objective estimation which can be recorded and compared with future reports of consumption.

The use of a retrospective drinking diary (Box 12.3) provides a record of alcohol consumption over a specific period of time, thus incorporating both the pattern and level of consumption. This should be recorded for the week immediately prior to the assessment and is achieved by asking the patient or client how much he or she drank on that particular day, the day before, the day before that, etc. It is likely that prompts will be required, such as 'Try to remember where you were and who you were with ...'. The responses should be recorded on a chart (Box 12.3) and kept in the patient or client's notes.[41]

If the previous week's consumption is found to exceed the recommended sensible limits, i.e. in excess of 21 standard drinks per week for males or 14 standard drinks for women, you should probe further using a standard questionnaire, such as the World Health Organization's Alcohol Use Disorders Identification Test (AUDIT)[31] (Box 12.4). Patients who score 8 or more on the AUDIT questionnaire should be advised to cut down their drinking.

An additional reason for making a detailed record of alcohol consumption is that helping patients or clients to consider their drinking in this way can, in itself, be an effective intervention which results in prompting problem drinkers to cut down their drinking to within sensible limits.[38]

Using the retrospective drinking diary and the AUDIT (see Boxes 12.3 and 12.4, respectively) has been shown to be a more reliable method for early identification of potential problem drinkers than using blood tests such as liver enzymes or mean cell volume.[42,43] However, blood concentrations of gamma glutamyltransferase (GGT) and aspartate transaminase (AST) rise progressively with alcohol intake and are more useful as indicators of relatively prolonged alcohol use.[44] Raised mean cell volume (MCV) can also be associated with excessive alcohol consumption.[44] It is therefore appropriate that a detailed drinking history should be taken from patients who are found to have raised levels of GGT and AST, and increased MCV.

Box 12.3 Retrospective diary of alcohol consumption

Complete the following chart indicating:

- *how much* alcohol you drank last week
- *what kind of alcohol* you had to drink (e.g. spirits, wine, beer – strong or low alcohol beer, etc.)
- *at what time of day* you were drinking.

Beginning with yesterday, work backwards through the week. If last week was *not* normal for you, think of what would be a typical week for you when filling in the chart.

	Morning	**Afternoon**	**Evening**
Monday			
Tuesday			
Wednesday			
Thursday			
Friday			
Saturday			
Sunday			

Total number of drinking days ....

Maximum amount consumed in 24 hours...

Total week's consumption ....

Advice

The large majority of individuals who are screened in the way described above will be low-risk drinkers for which no further action will be required. Those individuals who are found to be moderate drinkers should be taught how to calculate their consumption in 'standard drinks' of alcohol. Advice should be given about spreading their drinking throughout the week so that binge drinking is discouraged. On the other hand, it should be pointed out that everyone should have at least two 'alcohol-free' days each week.

Box 12.4 Audit [31]

Please circle the answer that is correct for you:

Q1: How often do you have a drink containing alcohol?
- Never   0
- Monthly   1
- Two to four times a month   2
- Two to three times a week   3
- Four or more times a week   4

Q2: How many drinks of alcohol do you have on a typical day when you are drinking?
- One or two   0
- Three or four   1
- Five or six   2
- Seven to nine   3
- Ten or more   4

Q3: How often do you have six or more drinks on one occasion?
- Never   0
- Less than monthly   1
- Monthly   2
- Weekly   3
- Daily or almost daily   4

Q4: How often during the last year were you unable to stop drinking once you had started?
- Never   0
- Less than monthly   1
- Monthly   2
- Weekly   3
- Daily or almost daily   4

Q5: How often during the last year did you fail to do what was normally expected from you because of drinking?
- Never   0
- Less than monthly   1
- Monthly   2
- Weekly   3
- Daily or almost daily   4

Q6: How often during the last year have you needed a first drink in the morning to get yourself going after a heavy drinking session?
- Never 0
- Less than monthly 1
- Monthly 2
- Weekly 3
- Daily or almost daily 4

Q7: How often during the last year have you had a feeling of guilt or remorse after drinking?
- Never 0
- Less than monthly 1
- Monthly 2
- Weekly 3
- Daily or almost daily 4

Q8: How often during the last year have you been unable to remember what happened the night before because you had been drinking?
- Never 0
- Less than monthly 1
- Monthly 2
- Weekly 3
- Daily or almost daily 4

Q9: Have you or someone else been injured as a result of your drinking?
- Never 0
- Yes, but not in the last year 2
- Yes, during the last year 4

Q10: Has a relative or friend, or doctor or other health professional been concerned about your drinking or suggested you cut down?
- No 0
- Yes, but not in the last year 2
- Yes, during the last year 4

Scoring
- Questions 1 to 3 total: male scoring > 4. female scoring > 3. Indicative of potential hazardous alcohol consumption.
- Questions 4 to 6 total: male or female scoring > 4. Indicative that there may be a level of dependency.
- All questions total: male or female scoring > 8. Indicative of potential hazardous alcohol consumption.
- All questions total: male or female scoring < 8. Indicative of consumption within safe limits.

People are more likely to change habits such as drinking if they recognise that there are benefits in doing so. For this reason it is helpful to encourage at-risk drinkers to draw up a 'balance sheet' of what are, for them, positive and negative effects of drinking. This can be done within a motivational interviewing framework and, by using 'active listening', can help the individual to focus on the effects of their drinking and to decide for themselves that they should change[45] (*see also* Chapter 13).

Such individuals should be reassured that they are not being advised to stop drinking, rather they should be encouraged to conclude for themselves that it is in their best interest to reduce consumption levels. By helping them to calculate their consumption in 'standard drinks' it will have become apparent that different alcoholic beverages contain different concentrations of alcohol. Therefore, by changing what they drink, for example a beer whose alcohol percentage volume is 5% to one of 3.5%, a reduction can be achieved relatively easily. Information should also be given about sensible drinking levels and health risks associated with increasing levels of consumption. Individuals should be encouraged to consider whether they drink in response to certain situations, or perhaps when in certain company. Encouraging problem drinkers to identify certain patterns or antecedents to drinking for themselves can also help them to work out alternative strategies for coping with these issues.

The information described above can be supplemented by giving health education literature which patients or clients can consult later in the privacy of their own home and in their own time. Such literature includes Health Education Authority (England) pamphlets such as *That's the limit: a guide to sensible drinking*.

Individuals who are found to be in the high-risk category should be referred for further assessment with a view to offering specialist treatment. They should also be offered self-help manuals such as *So you want to cut down your drinking?* which is produced by the Health Education Board (Scotland). This manual describes measures which can be adopted to help reduce consumption and gives details about how to use a drinking diary to calculate consumption and monitor drinking. It also gives information about a variety of treatment facilities in the individual's local area.

Education for professionals

In order for healthcare professionals to be able to assess levels of alcohol consumption accurately, they need to be able to measure this in a standard way as described earlier in this chapter. It is therefore important for them also to know the alcohol content of different beverages as well as the levels of consumption above which there is increasing risk of developing health problems.

Studies have shown that although there is general agreement among nurses that it is important that they ask patients about their alcohol consumption, few do so accurately.[46] They acknowledge that they have a role in providing guidance about sensible drinking, but many feel unsure about the nature of the information which they should be giving.[46,47] The majority of participants were unclear about the concept of the standard drink of alcohol and were unsure of the accepted sensible limits of alcohol consumption to enable them to provide this information to patients.[46,47] In Watson's study, most nurses did possess knowledge of a wide variety of alcohol-related health problems associated with prolonged drinking. However, most cited problems which are associated with dependence rather than those which are of value in detecting problem drinkers at an early stage.[46]

In both Cooper's[47] and Watson's[46] studies, the majority of participants recognised that it is appropriate for them to give advice to problem drinkers, but only a minority reported doing so in practice. They did not consider that they have been adequately trained to fulfil this role. In addition, alcohol-related health education literature was not available at ward level for the majority of nurses to give to patients.[46]

It is possible that these findings do not relate solely to nurses, but may reflect the position for members of other health professionals. The results of this study suggest that if nurses are to develop a role in the prevention of alcohol problems, the deficits in their education and practice need to be addressed. They need to become better informed about sensible drinking limits as well as early alcohol problems so that they can fulfil their patient education role. It may be that as alcohol problems have traditionally been treated within specialist psychiatric services, so the teaching of alcohol problems and treatments of such have remained the responsibility of specialist or psychiatric nurse teachers. However, alcohol problems affect almost every aspect of health. Teaching about the relationship between alcohol and health ought to be an integral part of the entire curriculum and be within the remit of all who teach about healthcare.

Conclusion

The measures outlined in this chapter are part of a spectrum of approach which can be used at both a population and individual level to prevent the occurrence of alcohol-related harm. Education is a powerful instrument both with which to raise public awareness of the relationship between alcohol and health, and also to equip those who have opportunities to promote sensible drinking.

To develop your knowledge in this area, see 'To learn more', p. 265.

Self-assessment questions

1 Whom does problem drinking affect?
2 How can success in reducing the amount of alcohol which *everyone* drinks help to reduce alcohol-related problems by a relatively greater proportion?
3 What are the Health Education Authority's recommended limits for sensible drinking?
4 (i)   One pint of 4.5% alcohol by volume (ABV) beer contains two standard drinks of alcohol. True or false?
  (ii) One can of extra-strong lager contains the equivalent of a double measure of whisky. True or false?
  (iii) One bottle of 8% ABV table wine contains six standard drinks of alcohol. True or false?
  (iv) One standard drink is contained in 25 ml of spirits. True or false?
5 How many alcohol-free days should everyone have each week?
6 Is it better to use a quantity and frequency measure or a retrospective diary to assess a person's level and pattern of alcohol consumption?

CHAPTER 13

New perspectives on motivation and change

Theresa B Moyers

Pre-reading exercise

Please take a moment to consider a change you will try to make in your own life within the next six months. Think of the reasons you would like to make the change, as well as reasons against it. Keep this situation in mind as you read the following chapter.

> 'I know I drink too much sometimes, but I'm not an alcoholic like my dad. Maybe if my wife would quit nagging me about it, I could cut down like I should.'
>
> Joe A. in a conversation with a treatment provider in an alcohol treatment programme

Joe's provider has a dilemma. He wants to persuade Joe to accept the need for a change in his drinking, and he is acutely aware of the risks Joe is taking and the likely outcome if he does not slow down or stop his drinking altogether. He feels an urgency for resolution and change, but he also sees that Joe is resistant, and he is wary of alienating him by pushing too hard. What will he do?

It is no exaggeration to say that this provider's dilemma reflects one of the central issues in alcohol treatment today. While the technology of treatment improves almost more rapidly than providers can keep up with it,[1,2] the ability to engage and motivate clients is more elusive. Fortunately, new models of motivating and engaging clients offer a fresh perspective on intervening with problem drinkers like Joe.

The stages-of-change model[3] represents behaviour change as a circular, continuous process rather than a single event. This change process is symbolised by a wheel, which has several stages through which people progress as they attempt to change a problematic behaviour (Figure 13.1). Progress to each succeeding stage is determined by events and decisions in the previous one.

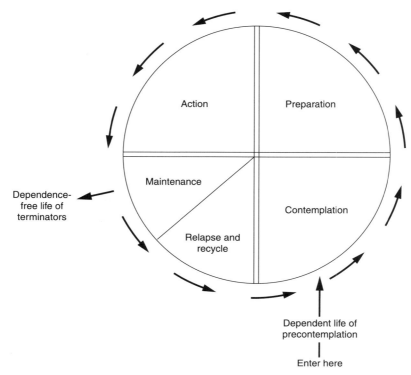

Figure 13.1 Stages of change in the cycle of change.[3]

The first stage, *precontemplation*, represents a state of surprise or resistance. Here, the person either is unaware of the need for change or has no intent to change. A client in this stage of change might be surprised that others are requesting a change from them. He may be annoyed that others are more concerned about his behaviour than he is. The provider's task for the client in precontemplation is to educate and raise awareness of the consequences of the problem behaviour.

It is important to note, however, that our hypothetical client, Joe, is not in this stage of change. He is aware of some consequences of his drinking and he does perceive a need to change, although he is conflicted about it. Joe represents an example of the contemplation stage of change, next in the wheel. A person in the *contemplation* stage is considering change, but has not yet endorsed it. The problem drinker in this stage is likely to be ambivalent, having both concerns about his drinking and a strong attachment to it. This ambivalence may be manifested as profound indecision and a contemplator may drive his treatment providers to distraction with a constant see-sawing about whether or not a change must be made. This ambivalence carries a trap for providers because when a client is transfixed between two sides of the equation for change, and is compelled to consider one side, the other is likely to become more attractive.[4] Providers who speak eloquently and logically about the need for change with a contemplator, therefore, may be unknowingly increasing the value of the *status quo*. The upshot of this is that the more the provider argues for change, the more resistant the client may become to it: a frustrating exchange, which has driven many clients and providers from each other in exasperation. What is needed to intervene more effectively with clients in the contemplation stage of change are specific techniques for negotiating and resolving ambivalence. Motivational interviewing, which will be discussed later in this chapter, is one method for doing just this.

At some point in the progress of contemplation, especially if the provider is skillful, the client may begin to prepare for change. *Preparation* is similar to a threshold the client passes through on the way to making a serious behaviour change. During preparation, the person may begin making small alterations (such as calling treatment programmes or counting the number of daily drinks) to experiment. Preparation, however, is transitory, for a person cannot comfortably stand for very long on a threshold.

After preparation the person enters the *action* stage of change. It is here that behaviour begins to change in a way that is visible and meaningful to others. Here is where providers are usually most comfortable in their work, and they typically offer a variety of strategies to assist clients in making these changes successfully. The action stage of change is often vibrant for both clients and providers; the client begins to experience the benefits of the behaviour change and feels some release from the pressure of problem drinking. The provider working with a client in the action stage of change typically feels a sense of satisfaction and excitement in their helping role.

Once the client successfully accomplishes a behaviour change (typically about six months) he enters the *maintenance* stage of change. Now the focus shifts from the acute crisis of breaking the dependence to the task of rearranging one's life to sustain the change. The provider assists the client to make specific changes, which result in a balance of life activities and reduce the chance of relapse.

Relapse is an event which terminates either action or maintenance. Once a relapse has occurred, the client may return to contemplation or may return directly to action. In the worst case scenario, the client may become completely demoralised and return to the precontemplation stage of change. The therapist's task when a relapse occurs is to assist the client in coping with disappointment and guilt so that the behaviour change process can be resumed.

Thus, in successfully making the transition out of a self-destructive behaviour, the client passes through a series of stages with specific characteristics. Ambivalence is considered a normal part of the change process; indeed, clients cannot begin to change without it. From this perspective, client ambivalence is not to be considered resistance, rather an expected product of transition. Within a stages-of-change model, resistance is provoked when the client is in the contemplation stage and the provider is in the action stage. Providers, committed to positive change and doing what they know best, may actually elicit resistance by using strategies for action with a highly ambivalent client. The provider's dilemma, again.

One important contribution of the stages-of-change model has been to redefine the provider's task, depending on the client's stage of change. Rather than advocate for immediate change, the provider must assess the client's stage of change and offer stage-appropriate interventions. When the provider has discovered that the client is ambivalent, he may choose strategies which reduce ambivalence and decrease resistance rather than inviting the client to action.

Motivational interviewing[5] is precisely such an approach. It is a therapeutic strategy for helping clients resolve ambivalence and increase their own innate motivation for change. Motivational interviewing (MI) is most useful for clients in the contemplation stage of change, but may be used for those who are ambivalent or resistant in any stage of change. The spirit of motivational interviewing is one of collaboration, so providers using this approach view their clients as capable and autonomous. They understand that persuasion has limited value and that their clients are the only ones who can choose to make a behaviour change. Therapists using this approach view their clients as the experts in making any change for themselves. They understand that the client's own values and goals provide the most potent source of motivation for change.

Within an MI approach, the therapist will refrain from advocating *for* change, understanding that this may cause an ambivalent client to become more attached to the option of *not* changing. Instead, the therapist structures the interview in ways that ensure that the client is the one presenting the arguments for change. The client should, in effect, talk himself into change by making self-motivational statements. The therapist's role is to arrange the interview so that the client has the best chance of making these statements. In attempting to do this, the provider is guided by five basic principles (Box 13.1).

The first principle is to *express empathy*, which indicates the importance of an engaged and empathic provider. In the treatment outcome literature for problem drinking, provider empathy is consistently powerful in predicting client outcomes, sometimes even more important than variables such as the type or amount of treatment received.[6] The definition of

Box 13.1 Five principles of motivational interviewing[5]

1 Express empathy
2 Develop discrepancy
3 Avoid argumentation
4 Roll with resistance
5 Support self-efficacy

empathy here is specific: it is the ability of the provider to accurately reflect what the client is saying. Providers who offer accurate reflections consistently and frequently during sessions with problem drinkers have better outcomes and are perceived as being empathic by their clients.[7–9] Empathy within an MI framework does not mean feeling sympathy for clients, having had the same experiences as clients or agreeing with them. Instead, it is defined as the ability to employ active listening skills.

The second principle for using motivational interviewing is to *develop discrepancy*. This indicates the importance of the client's most deeply held values and goals as a source of motivation for change. Providers are encouraged to find out what is most important to clients, what they hope for in the future and to explore the client's value system. When clients are too demoralised to discuss their hopes, it may be useful to ask what was important to them in the most satisfying time of their life. The gap, or discrepancy, between what clients hold most dear and their current drinking is the location of fruitful therapeutic work. It is the provider's goal to gently make that discrepancy explicit.

The third principle of motivational interviewing is to *avoid argumentation*. This indicates the importance of keeping resistance to a minimum by avoiding outright conflict with clients. The provider declines the expert role and invites the client's perspective. The provider is encouraged to place a higher value on decreasing resistance than on any particular detail of the diagnosis or recovery plan, unless there are insurmountable ethical obstacles.

The fourth principle of motivational interviewing is to *roll with resistance*. This indicates the value of meeting resistance with reflection rather than confrontation, and allowing clients to 'win their point' in disputes. It creates an obligation for the provider to be creative and flexible when resistance is encountered, and avoid power struggles. Clients are sometimes even encouraged to disregard what the provider is saying, choosing for themselves whether details apply to their own situation.

The last principle of motivational interviewing is to *support self-efficacy*. This indicates that clients must believe that they can make a specific behaviour change, like abstinence or moderate intake, in order for it to happen. The provider looks for opportunities to encourage the client in honest ways, and affirm their chances of being successful. When clients are pessimistic, the provider looks hard for other successes and strengths in the client's life to support the notion that they can make this change as well.

In using motivational interviewing, the provider will begin with five basic skills which are guided by the principles discussed above. The first four of these skills are borrowed from general clinical practice and are not specific to MI, so they will not be discussed in detail. However, it is important to note that these skills, especially reflective listening, are not merely a *part* of motivational interviewing but the essential foundation for it. The provider using motivational interviewing will:

1 ask open-ended questions
2 listen reflectively
3 affirm
4 summarise periodically
5 (specific to MI) elicit self-motivational statements.

Self-motivational statements are comments by the client indicating a need or desire for change, for example 'I don't want my drinking to ruin my life the way it did my father's'. It is the provider's task to arrange the interview so that the client makes such statements. This is important not simply so that the interview will be congenial, but because clients are more likely to believe such statements when they speak them, rather than hear them from someone else.[10]

In eliciting self-motivational statements the provider may draw from a variety of approaches, choosing which seems best depending on the client's resistance and level of interest. A provider might engage in a decisional balance exercise in which the pros and cons of both changing and not changing are formally listed. An ambivalent client might be asked to discuss what are the very best things about drinking and what he would miss most about it. The interviewer might ask the client to envision his life in five years, perhaps choosing to ask what differences he might see if he were not drinking. A values clarification exercise in which the client is asked to be specific and give examples of the values most important to him could be an option[11] (Box 13.2). The guiding principle behind eliciting self-motivational statements is that the interviewer should facilitate the client's self-expression of desire or intent to change. In general, the interview should proceed along this course, with the interviewer encouraging the client to consider their deepest goals and values in life and to explore whatever innate motivation is already present for a change.

Box 13.2 Approaches to eliciting self-motivational changes

Provider: an individual providing substance abuse screening, assessment or treatment.

Decisional balance exercise: an activity in which the client and the provider generate both the pros and cons of changing a behaviour as well as the pros and cons of the *status quo*.

Values clarification exercise: an activity in which the client is asked to sort or prioritise his or her own values from a larger pool of possible values.

Note: Please note that the above are generic, rather than specific, terms. For example, the values clarification exercise described by Rokeach[11] is only one example of a value exercise.

To elicit self-motivational statements, the interviewer might also ask particular kinds of questions which seem likely to 'pull' for self-motivational answers. From the example above, the provider might ask 'What do you see about your drinking that reminds you of your father's?' Evocative questions might be asked about the client's concern about his drinking, the manner in which he recognises it as a problem (or not), the ways he has thought about changing and what hope he has about accomplishing a change. Providers are guided by the five principles of MI (see Box 13.1) in forming such questions, and may avoid them altogether if it seems they will increase resistance.

If resistance, or counter-motivational behaviour, is encountered, the interviewer should do what is necessary, within acceptable therapeutic practice, to decrease it so that the proper work of revealing and enhancing implicit motivation can proceed. The interviewer adheres to the principles of avoiding argumentation and rolling with resistance in specific ways. Simple reflections of the client's meaning and emotion are the approach of choice when clients are hostile or the interviewer is uncertain. Other approaches might include reflections that slightly exaggerate the client's point of view (an amplified reflection) or offer both sides of the ambivalence that is being offered (a double-sided reflection). An example of a double-sided reflection for Joe A., our hypothetical client at the beginning of the chapter, might go something like this: 'So on the one hand you feel like you might be drinking too much, but on the other hand you resent it when your wife pushes you toward quitting.' Interviewers may also consider agreeing with the client that they alone can make the decision to change and cannot be forced to do so against their will (emphasising personal choice and control). If the collaboration between the interviewer and the client is good, the interviewer might choose to respond to resistance by voicing arguments against change, with the goal of eliciting the opposite point of view. At all times, the interviewer is monitoring his own emotional tone, falling back on simple reflections when feelings of irritation, anger or exasperation toward client resistance are discovered. This is crucial, since any of the MI techniques for responding to counter-motivational behaviour can be destructive if they are offered in a sarcastic or punitive manner. In general, the guiding principle in responding to resistance is to avoid any sort of power struggle which will exacerbate it, and thereby decrease the probability of positive behaviour change.

If motivational interviewing works well, the therapeutic interaction should culminate in meaningful self-motivational statements from the client and little evidence of resistance toward change. At this point, the interviewer may want to shift direction and begin to explicitly ask the client to consider making a change. This is done through the use of key questions. For example the interviewer might summarise all the reasons the client has given both for and against change and then ask the client 'Where does this leave you?' or 'What do you make of all this?' or any other question which gently opens the door toward movement and is appropriate. If the client is willing to make a commitment to change at that time, then the therapist might begin working to form a joint treatment plan or to discuss possible solutions for specific roadblocks the client faces. If the client remains ambivalent, the interviewer might invite the client to continue the process of examining options using an MI format or to return in the future if the picture changes.

Motivational interviewing is a specific therapeutic approach to working with substance-abusing clients and can be used in a variety of ways. Empirical evidence indicates that MI can enhance client outcomes when it is used prior to traditional treatments,[12,13] perhaps by assisting clients to resolve ambivalence and become more receptive to the help they encounter. But motivational interviewing is also effective as a brief, stand-alone intervention in lieu of other treatments,[14] perhaps assisting clients to harness the power of their own motivation and make changes without the help of providers.

Motivational interviewing enhances the continuum of care for substance abuse problems, and provides effective options for patients who are not yet committed to engage in the change process.[15] The manner in which it can be incorporated in any particular setting will depend on the treatment culture, the needs of the patients and the clinical judgement of the providers as well as the resources available for funding treatment options. Finally, it is clear that motivational interviewing is a learnable skill. Several rigorous studies have been completed in which therapists new to MI were taught to use it and carefully supervised with excellent evidence of employing it well.[16] Nevertheless, not all were able to do so. Motivational interviewing, like every other therapeutic intervention, fares better with some providers than with others.[17] In general, it is easier for providers to use MI well when they have a solid foundation in clinical skills, have learned to avoid power struggles with their clients and can view human behaviour change as a complex process in which they have a small part to play.

To develop your knowledge in this area, see 'To learn more', p. 266.

Post-reading exercise

Consider the change you selected at the beginning of the chapter. Can you place yourself in the stages-of-change wheel? Do you recognise any ambivalence about making this change? Considering the motivational interviewing approach described above, what is your next step?

Self-assessment questions

1 Motivational interviewing is a therapeutic technique for clients who:
   (a) are determined not to change their drinking habits
   (b) are already making changes in their drinking habits
   (c) need intensive in-patient care to make a change in their drinking habits
   (d) are ambivalent about making changes in their drinking habits

2 When using motivational interviewing, a therapist will respond to resistance with:
   (a) confrontation
   (b) information
   (c) reflection
   (d) logic

3 In outcome research, motivational interviewing has been shown to be useful as:
   (a) an enhancement prior to traditional treatment
   (b) an example of a Minnesota model intervention
   (c) a stand-alone treatment
   (d) a and c

4 When clients are ambivalent about changing, providers using motivational interviewing should:
(a) avoid giving advice so that resistance is not provoked
(b) avoid being timid and confront the ambivalence directly
(c) convey empathy by telling clients of their own experiences
(d) remind the client of the consequences of their drinking

5 A client who has stopped drinking for two months, is keeping regular appointments with the therapist and avoiding risky situations for relapse is in what stage of change:
(a) contemplation
(b) action
(c) preparation
(d) maintenance

CHAPTER 14

Essentials of assessment

Pip Mason

Learning outcomes

This chapter will assist the reader in being able to:

- describe the purpose and aims of assessment
- identify key questions and areas of enquiry for an assessment in a given context
- describe the ways in which counselling skills can improve the process of an assessment.

What is assessment?

Assessment is an exchange of information. The information is used to plan goals and interventions. Howard and colleagues have described it as 'the foundation of case management'.[1]

It can be seen as an ongoing process. In one sense assessment begins even before either the worker or the client identifies that alcohol is an issue to address. Then, having made a provisional plan, continuous assessment takes place to ensure interventions are adjusted to best meet the client's needs.

However, there is usually a point when the worker formally sits down with the drinker (and with their family or significant others) and systematically puts together the information required to decide on the exact nature of the problem and how best to move forward.

Grant and Hodgson,[2] in their manual for primary healthcare workers, describe the main aims of assessment of substance use problems as:

- 'to obtain as much accurate information as possible about the individual's drug use and any associated problems'
- 'to try to identify the factors associated with drug abuse in the individual – these may be physical illnesses, or social or psychological problems'
- 'to assist the worker in identifying the strengths and weaknesses of the individual and his or her family, as well as their ability to cope with, and assist in the management of, the problem'.

Why is assessment important?

Heavy drinking does not take place in isolation. It is a response to, or a cause of, other problems. Social, legal, economic, emotional, physical, developmental, spiritual and creative aspects of a person's life can be affected by drinking. Other people may also become involved and have a stake in the heavy drinker changing.

The solutions to such problems usually lie in the drinker changing their behaviour. People whose drinking causes them difficulties have to be the main agents of change (*see also* Chapter 13). The worker's role, even if it also includes some highly technical aspects, is primarily to facilitate self-help. Consequently, in order to make a plan it is necessary to have good information about the drinker's inclinations, strengths and abilities as well as about their problems and difficulties. The question is not so much 'What shall I do?' but 'What can he or she do and how can I help?'.

What should an assessment include?

The content of an assessment is a difficult issue. The best answer is 'it depends ...'. It is only possible to decide what information you need when you have clarified why you need it and what you are going to do with it. Ask yourself the following questions in relation to the assessments that you do in your own work.

- What are the decisions we each and or both have to make (i.e. you and your client)?
- What information do we need to help us make these decisions?

The following examples illustrate the way the content of an assessment may vary.

EXAMPLE 1 (SELF-ASSESSMENT EXERCISE)
A primary care nurse identifies that a patient is drinking more than double the recommendations for low-risk drinking.

The decisions to be made:

Client: Do I want to do anything about it?
Nurse: Do I intervene to try to reduce this patient's drinking? Shall I refer them to someone else?

1 What information do you think needs to be collected to help the patient make these decisions together?
2 List some key questions.

Compare your list with the following.

Together, they need to explore:

- Is the current pattern of drinking causing any problems?
- What problems might it cause if this pattern continues?
- To what extent is the *patient* concerned about these actual or potential problems?
- To what extent is the *nurse* concerned about these actual or potential problems?
- Does the patient want to change? If so, how difficult will it be? Will any other help be needed (e.g. detoxification, a structured programme for reducing drinking, peer support)?
- Has the patient tried to change in the past? If so, what has been helpful before? What can be learned from past attempts?
- If the patient does not want to change, does the nurse have responsibilities to intervene in any other problems related to the drinking (e.g. child neglect or abuse)? Is there any scope for harm reduction (e.g. vitamin supplements to improve nutritional status)?

Compare this with another example from a different context.

EXAMPLE 2 (SELF-ASSESSMENT EXERCISE)
A counsellor in a specialist alcohol agency has a first appointment with a client who has referred herself because she is frightened. She feels she is losing control over her drinking.

The decisions to be made:

Client: Shall I embark on a course of counselling at this agency?
Counsellor: Shall I take this person on for counselling? Should I refer her elsewhere for additional or alternative help?

1 What information do you think needs to be collected or shared to help them to make these decisions?
2 Make another list of key questions or issues for an assessment in this context.

Compare your list with the following suggestions of key issues.

The client needs to understand:

- what sort of counselling is available and how it might be expected to help her. She also needs to know what level of commitment (time, cost, willingness to talk about intimate issues) it will entail.

The counsellor needs to understand:

- the nature and history of the presenting alcohol problem
- other related problems, including use of other drugs
- previous attempts to change and outcome
- present circumstances – home, employment, health
- immediate needs
- any problems that would interfere with the client making use of counselling (e.g. psychiatric, psychological or neuropsychological)
- the client's beliefs about drinking and drink problems
- the client's feelings about the prospect of change; how important is it to her to change and how confident does she feel about being able to do so.

In Example 1 the assessment priorities are related to *health problems* because of the setting, and *readiness to change* because the nurse has only just identified the issue. Consideration of treatment options followed on from these primary issues.

In Example 2 the priorities are to identify *whether counselling might help* and *other help required*. Although, of course, health and readiness to change are still relevant issues, the client has already provisionally decided drinking is a problem and she wants to seek help. The immediate issue now is what sort of help to arrange for her.

Mattick and Jarvis'[3] quality assurance review (1994) recommends that assessment for specialist intervention should:

> *'provide information about the client's consumption of alcohol, level of alcohol dependence, cognitive functioning, psychological co-morbidity, family situation, physical well-being and readiness for change.'*

In any given situation the worker will decide which of these to explore in most depth. In a primary care setting the family situation, general health profile and social circumstances may already be known. It will therefore be appropriate to concentrate mainly on the specifics of the drinking. Specialists in secondary or tertiary care agencies often start with very limited information and need to ask about the broader picture.

Assessing the drinking

A baseline is needed in order to plan change. It is necessary to establish 'What is it about the drinking that is problematic?'. Frequently the quantity, frequency and consequent intoxication, in themselves, cause the problems. Sometimes, however, less heavy drinking is nevertheless problematic because of the context (e.g. at work or college or when driving). Others find their drinking problematic because of their own feelings about it (e.g. someone whose drinking is incompatible with their religious beliefs or with their self-image).

The following questions form a useful structure for understanding the drinking in context.

What is the client's drinking pattern?
- What do they drink and under what circumstances?
- How much?
- How frequently?
- Where?
- At what times of the day?
- With whom?
- Do they use any other drugs and, if so, how does this fit in with the drinking?

History
- How does this compare with the way the client has drunk in the past?
- Does the client connect periods of increased drinking with any particular events or feelings?
- Has the client tried to reduce or stop drinking previously? If so, what happened?

Problems
- Does the drinking cause, or make worse, any problems?
- Problems the client has noticed?
- Any other problems, which are not seen by the client as necessarily alcohol-related?

The functions drinking has in the person's life
- What does the client get from drinking?
- With what situations does it help them cope?

Readiness to change
- As the client sees it, what are the pros and cons of drinking?
- Is the client:
  - content to continue the current pattern of drinking?
  - wondering sometimes about cutting down or stopping?
  - keen to stop or cut down as soon as possible?
  - at risk of relapsing, having already cut down or stopped?

Prospects for the future
- What are the implications (good and bad) of the client changing his or her drinking:
  - for the client?
  - for the family?
  - for anyone else?

Beliefs about drink problems
- How does the client view drinking problems?
- How does he or she see their own drinking fitting into this?
- What sort of 'treatment' or 'intervention' does he or she believe to be useful in helping people with such difficulties?

Clearly the frameworks discussed in the previous chapter for understanding the stages of change and ways to engage motivation are useful in the assessment stage (*see* Chapter 13). A full assessment includes identifying the positive functions of drinking, as well as the problems related to it. The client's views of, and feelings about, it are important as well as the objective facts about the behaviour. The information collected about the drinking *pattern* is important in assessing whether the client is likely to experience withdrawal symptoms if they stop drinking suddenly. If someone is drinking every day, drinking first thing in the morning and wants to stop drinking, it is worth considering detoxification (*see* Chapter 15).

Assessing problems associated with the drinking

Investigation of related problems is important and the way this is done will vary according to the context of the assessment. A doctor or nurse will have particular responsibilities and facilities to check on liver function, blood pressure and general health issues. A probation officer will be most concerned to help the client consider links between drinking and offending. Social workers will perhaps prioritise the effect the client's drinking has on the rest of the family and his or her ability to fulfil family responsibilities. In the workplace a key focus will be the effect of drinking and hangovers on work performance and safety. When the client is reluctant to discuss the drinking, it is easiest if all enquiries into alcohol problems are seen as 'legitimate', i.e. that they are clearly within the worker's remit.

Self-assessment exercise

If you work in a non-specialist setting it may be worth asking yourself: 'In what ways is it my business to ask about people's drinking? Isn't it their own affair how much they drink?' Try making a list of ways in which people's drinking impinges upon the aspects of their lives which *are* your business. Do this from the perspective of your own job before moving on.

Having done that it will probably be clear to you that sometimes it is impossible for you to do your job properly and help with the presenting problems without bringing drinking into the picture. In discussing the drinking it is usually best to start with these areas, which you and the client can both see are directly relevant to the other matters in hand. By doing so it is easier to be matter of fact and orientated towards problem solving. Talk about the effects and functions of the drinking: 'Do you think that drinking helps you to…?' or 'Do you think there is any connection between the fact that you enjoy a drink and…?' rather than attempting to apply labels, as in: 'Would you call yourself a heavy drinker?' or 'Have you ever thought you might be alcoholic?' On the other hand, it helps if a rounded picture of the client and the drinking can be built up eventually. A holistic view of the issue can be taken, once rapport and trust are established.

The process of assessment

The style and the tools used for assessment vary between organisations and between practitioners. In specialist agencies the assessment may be the first encounter between the client and the therapist or counsellor. In a non-specialist setting, assessment of the drinking may be the first in-depth discussion about alcohol, although there may be an existing therapeutic relationship with other foci. The *way* the assessment is conducted and the way the information is collected will influence the rapport between worker and client, which in turn will affect the process of any interventions that follow. Hyams *et al.*[4] examined clients' experiences of, and satisfaction with, the assessment interview in a therapeutic day unit, and their subsequent engagement (or not) in treatment. They found that clients who reported a 'positive therapeutic relationship' with the worker were more likely to engage than clients who reported a negative experience. The clients most likely to engage were those who felt the worker to be 'warm, accepting, understanding and knowledgeable' and to 'genuinely want to work with them'.

Clancy and Coyne[5] highlight the need for assessment to take place in a safe, confidential environment, with sensitivity towards issues of race, culture, gender, sexuality, religion and age (*see also* Chapter 10). Hyams *et al.*[4] found clients commented positively on the workers' 'understanding of the real me' and 'ability to understand my personal situation and problems'. So the structure of the assessment needs to allow for development of a good relationship. Mattick and Jarvis[3] recommended a 'semi-structured, narrative style' which culminates in 'a summary of the facts and a formulation of a clear, mutually acceptable treatment plan that structures a specific intervention to meet the needs of the individual'.

For some people assessment is all that is wanted or needed. It provides an opportunity to gain an insight into the way drinking is interacting with other aspects of their lives and to reflect on the pros and cons of changing. This can be the catalyst for changes with which the client can proceed unaided. The information collected should be at least as useful to the client as it is to the worker. A summary and feedback can facilitate this. Any subsequent plans for intervention or treatment can then be jointly made on the basis of a shared understanding.

Assessment tools and instruments

Apart from a 'good pair of ears' and a willingness to try to understand the drinking from the client's viewpoint, some pencil-and-paper exercises and questionnaires have been found to be useful.

Drink diary

The most common exercise, which clients can be taught to use, is a drink diary (Box 14.1). Most people for whom drinking is a part of their everyday life have no clear idea how much they drink. If asked to recall daily consumption in the previous week they cannot be entirely accurate because they were not counting at the time!

Keeping a record of consumption for a week (quantity, type of drink, time of day, company, venue) can provide a drinker with interesting insights. Frequently people find they drink more than they had initially thought. Sometimes they find that problematic drinking is associated with being in particular situations or in particular company. Calculating weekly expenditure on alcohol can be a motivating factor for some. Some people find that recording their mood before and after drinking throws light on the part alcohol plays in their life.

Many health promotion leaflets and self-help booklets on alcohol have a drink diary form in them. Alternatively it is easy to draw out a form, adding any columns that may be relevant or of interest to the individual (see Box 14.1). If the client has learned to calculate consumption in standard drinks this can be added, or the worker can help them do this later.

Box 14.1 shows how, for this client, the diary identifies that the heaviest drinking occurs when he goes out alone to his local pub, the Rose and Crown, and when he is drinking generally 'with the crowd' rather than with a specific companion. This might prompt him to explore further why this drinking is different and whether the 'Rose and Crown' drinking might need to be the primary focus for thinking about change.

Box 14.1 Drink diary example

DAY	WHEN?	WHERE?	WHAT?	WITH WHOM?	STANDARD DRINKS TOTAL FOR DAY
MONDAY	Evening	Rose & Crown	6 pints bitter	The crowd in the bar	12
TUESDAY	Lunchtime Evening	Rose & Crown At home	4 pints bitter 6 cans lager	Alone Father	20
WEDNESDAY	Evening	Queen's Head	2 pints bitter	Girlfriend	4
THURSDAY	Evening	Rose & Crown	10 pints bitter	The crowd in the bar	20
FRIDAY	Lunchtime Evening	Rose & Crown Rose & Crown	4 pints bitter 10 pints bitter	Work mates The crowd in the bar	28
SATURDAY	Evening	Restaurant	1 pint bitter 1 bottle wine 2 brandies	Girlfriend	11
SUNDAY	Lunchtime	Rose & Crown	3 pints bitter	Father	6
			STANDARD DRINKS TOTAL		101

A typical day

Instead of asking about a whole week's drinking, it can also be helpful to ask, in some detail, about a typical day. This is one of the strategies described in Rollnick and colleagues' *Brief Motivational Interviewing*.[6] Getting the client to take you through their day, from waking until bedtime, shows how the alcohol use fits into their other activities, moods and beliefs about how to cope with everyday stressors. It can help both the worker and the drinker to see more clearly what the drinking is about, and helps build rapport and mutual understanding.

Questionnaires and psychometric tests

Lettieri *et al.*[7] reviews 45 screening and diagnostic instruments, many of which are very detailed questionnaires or psychometric tests. Since Lettieri wrote in 1985, many more have been developed. The value of collecting such detailed information in such a highly structured way needs to be balanced against the risk of alienating the client and reducing the chance of them turning up for future counselling or treatment. Attempts to use the results of scientific assessments to match suitable treatments to clients with particular characteristics have not yet been very fruitful[8] so it seems important not to compromise the quality of the therapeutic relationship by using any questionnaires that are unnecessarily cumbersome.

However, where specific information is required and can be easily gained in the context of a client-centred interview, some questionnaires have been found by clinicians to be very valuable. For example, the Severity of Alcohol Dependence Questionnaire[9] (SADQ) is recommended by Cooper[10] for assessing whether to arrange home detoxification. Raistrick *et al.* have developed a 10-item self-completion questionnaire, the Leeds Dependence Questionnaire (LDQ)[11], which measures dependence on a variety of substances. It is sensitive to change over time so can be used to collect baseline information and then monitor the effectiveness of subsequent interventions.

Some clients enjoy completing questionnaires (provided they are 'user-friendly') and find feedback from the results helpful in clarifying the severity or nature of their problems. Others can explain their situation and their needs better through talking and telling stories to illustrate points. The assessor's skill is in eliciting the most accurate information possible and organising it in a way that helps all concerned to see a way forward.

How can you assess someone who won't tell you the truth?

People with drink problems are often suspected of concealing the truth about their drinking. Some do, of course. Helping people feel able to be honest is a skill, and one not restricted to working with drinkers. Some people recommend collecting corroborating evidence of some sort. The most common sources are family members (or significant others) and results of medical tests.

Families can be a part of the solution, and are sometimes a part of the problem. Involving them in the assessment can be very useful if the setting is appropriate. There are, of course, difficulties if one person's description of the problem is at odds with another's. It is not necessarily always the drinker who is giving a false picture. Sometimes even when everyone is being honest about how they see things, their accounts differ. Non-specialists often have skills in dealing with such difficulties in families, with regard to other problems. These skills will need to be brought into play in working with alcohol problems too.

Discussion of the results of medical tests, such as gamma glutamyl transferase (GGT) or mean corpuscular volume (MCV), is important and can add to the assessment picture. However, confronting the individual with such 'evidence' is not always the best way of dealing with a defensive, insecure drinker who does not yet feel safe enough to tell the truth. In the interest of developing a good therapeutic relationship in the future, it is best to work hard at helping the client feel safe, respected and cared about so that he or she will be honest, rather than waiting for him or her to lie and then be confronted with evidence of deceit! In the previous chapter resistance is discussed and a 'motivational interviewing' approach is most useful in enabling honesty (*see* Chapter 13). For most drinkers, drinking has benefits and helps them cope with certain situations. If the assessor is willing to listen to this side of the equation as well as compiling a problem list, a better rapport will be built.

Conclusion

The nature of an assessment needs to vary to suit the context. The prime focus will be the drinking itself, but this will need to be understood in the context of the client's life, circumstances, beliefs and values. Rather than seeing assessment as the worker collecting information and forming clinical judgements about the client, it is more accurate to think of the client and the worker jointly assessing the problem and considering possible solutions. The assessment process is not a neutral process. It is in itself an intervention and, if it is conducted well, can contribute considerably to the client's decision to embark on an action plan.

To develop your knowledge in this area, see 'To learn more', p. 268.

Self-assessment questions

1 Should assessment always be done by a specialist?
2 What do you think the difference is between screening and assessment?
3 What factors influence how successful the assessor is in getting truthful information from the client?
4 In what ways can an assessment process be helpful to the drinker?
5 In your work context, what are the aims of an assessment?

CHAPTER 15

Detoxification

Anne E Bartu

Pre-reading exercise

For one week, stop using your favourite substance, e.g. tea, coffee, alcohol, chocolate, tobacco. Each day, and at the end of the week, make a few notes on the following:

- How easy did you find it to live without your substance?
- Was your mood affected? If so, in what way? Did you experience craving or any other symptoms?
- What strategies did you use to avoid using your favourite substance? What worked and what didn't?

Detoxification has been defined as the management of the withdrawal reaction that occurs when a person who has been using psychoactive drugs, at a level which induces neuroadaptation and dependence, ceases use.[1] A psychoactive drug is one which, when consumed, has the capacity to modify the perceptions, mood, cognitive behaviour or motor function of the user. The drug most commonly used for this purpose is alcohol. Neuroadaptation is the altered sensitivity of cells and physiological responses that develop with repeated use of a drug, and withdrawal involves reversal of this process. Hence the signs and symptoms of the withdrawal syndrome are opposite to the effects of the drug concerned. For example, alcohol is a central nervous system (CNS) depressant, and withdrawal from the drug is characterised by CNS hyperactivity. Fundamental to understanding the withdrawal syndromes are the concepts of tolerance and dependence. Tolerance is a reduced sensitivity to a drug following repeated consumption.[2] This means that higher doses of a particular drug are required to obtain the effect previously achieved with smaller doses. Dependence has been defined as a state of adaptation to a drug, which may be psychological and or physical, which includes a compulsion to use the drug to experience its effects and avoid withdrawal symptoms.[2]

Alcohol withdrawal syndrome

The alcohol withdrawal syndrome is characterised by a wide range of symptoms (Box 15.1), none of which are specific to alcohol, and which occur in clusters.

Box 15.1 Signs and symptoms of the alcohol withdrawal syndrome

tremors	diarrhoea
muscle jerks	diaphoresis
increased heart rate	insomnia
elevated temperature	nightmares
hypertension	minor and major seizures
hyperventilation	hallucinations
anorexia	anxiety
nausea	depression
vomiting	delirium tremens

The withdrawal symptoms from alcohol include tremors, muscle jerks, increased heart rate, elevated temperature and blood pressure, hyperventilation, anorexia, nausea, vomiting, diarrhoea, diaphoresis, insomnia, nightmares, minor and major seizures, visual and auditory disturbances, peripheral neuritis, anxiety, depression and disorientation, and delirium tremens (DTs).[3]

These symptoms vary in severity and not all people will experience all symptoms. Mild withdrawal may involve no more than tremor, nausea, perspiration and restlessness. More severe forms, however, will include the full range of symptoms. The main complications are seizures and DTs. Seizures are usually singular and generalised. If they occur they most likely do so within the first 48 hours after drinking has stopped, and a single seizure usually requires little care and no medication. Delirium tremens, however, is a medical emergency that requires prompt treatment. The features of DTs are hallucinations, impaired attention and memory, disorientation and agitation. The withdrawal syndrome, in a severe form, can be life threatening.[3]

Onset of withdrawal symptoms

The onset of withdrawal symptoms from any psychoactive drug is related to the half-life of the drug. The shorter the half-life of a particular drug, the quicker the onset of withdrawal symptoms. For alcohol, these symptoms usually occur from six to 24 hours after the last intake of alcohol at customary levels. That is, when the blood alcohol concentration (BAC) approaches or reaches zero. It is not necessary for a person's BAC to reach zero before they start experiencing withdrawal symptoms. In some instances withdrawal symptoms may commence before all traces of alcohol are eliminated from the body.

Duration of withdrawals

Withdrawal symptoms are transient, vary in intensity and variety and last from two to 12 days. The more severe the symptoms, the longer the withdrawal episode. However, the duration and severity of withdrawal symptoms are difficult to predict because they are influenced by several interacting factors.[3] These include the frequency and duration of use of alcohol, other drug use, the nutritional status of the user, concomitant illness, the environment in which detoxification occurs and the expectations of the person concerned of the withdrawal process. For example, people who have experienced severe withdrawals are often apprehensive about the process, and are likely to become increasingly anxious and require considerable support to allay their fears.

The average length of the alcohol withdrawal syndrome is from three to five days, but some of the associated symptoms may persist for much longer. For example, with regard to sleep, specific abnormalities such as disturbances in rapid eye movement have been described which can be long lasting, and abnormal sleep electronencephalograms (EEGs) have been reported for up to 21 months after detoxification.[4]

Those at risk

People with a regular alcohol intake of 80–100 grams (8–10 standard drinks per day) or more should be considered to be at risk of withdrawing in the event that they abruptly reduce consumption. Ten grams of alcohol is approximately equal to one standard drink (*see also* Chapter 2). The severity of withdrawals is likely to be increased if a person has:

- had previous severe withdrawals
- co-morbidity, such as epilepsy, hypertension, cardiomyopathy, hepatitis, pancreatitis, pneumonia or a psychiatric condition.[5]

Assessment

Adequate assessment is essential to obtain information on which to make predictions about the likely nature and course of the withdrawal process. Assessment should include a history of the:

- quantity, frequency and duration of alcohol use
- time of the last drink
- use of other drugs, prescribed and non-prescribed
- previous withdrawal episodes
- medical conditions (epilepsy, hypertension, pancreatitis, blood-borne viruses, peptic ulcer, trauma, peripheral neuropathy, liver disease) and psychiatric conditions (schizophrenia, affective disorders, anxiety, psychosis, suicidal ideation, previous psychological treatment, etc.)
- social stressors (legal, relationships, job, financial problems)
- breathalyser reading
- level of dependence on alcohol.

An instrument that has been designed to measure alcohol dependence is the Severity of Alcohol Dependence Questionnaire (SADQ).[6] This instrument measures both physical and affective symptoms of withdrawal. The signs and symptoms of withdrawal, however, are related to the quantity, frequency and duration of alcohol consumption and opinion is divided on whether it is necessary to routinely include a measure of dependency in the assessment of people for detoxification. While some idea of dependence will alert health professionals to the possibility of withdrawal, when a person has presented for detoxification it may be sufficient to monitor progress on a standardised withdrawal scale.[7]

Management

The pathogenesis and pathophysiology of the alcohol withdrawal syndrome are complex. However, the management of it is relatively simple and is based on monitoring, supportive care and pharmacotherapy.

Monitoring

Monitoring involves assessing the client on a regular basis to determine the:

- severity of withdrawal symptoms
- need for medication
- nutritional status and fluid intake
- comfort.

Monitoring of withdrawal symptoms is best done with a standardised, well-validated, withdrawal scale. There are several such scales available. One that has been well validated is the revised Clinical Institute for Withdrawal Assessment for Alcohol (CIWA-AR).[8] The scale has 10 items that allow a quantitative assessment of the common withdrawal symptoms on a range of 0–7, with a maximum score of 67. Scores of <10 = mild withdrawal, 10–20 = moderate withdrawal, and 20+ = severe withdrawal. High scores on one or two items such as anxiety or hallucinations would indicate that further treatment was required, even if the overall score was <10. Another scale is the Symptom Severity Checklist.[7] The maximum score on this scale is 36, and a score of 18+ is cause for concern. Whatever scale is adopted will depend on the preference of the practitioner and ease of use with the client. It is important to remember that no withdrawal scale is a substitute for clinical judgement, and any cut-off point should best be regarded as a guideline and interpreted on the basis of clinical assessment.

Decisions about the frequency and duration of assessment are based on clinical judgement (Box 15.2). In general, monitoring may only be necessary on a second-hourly basis for the first day and fourth-hourly on the second day. Using the scale provides an opportunity to reassure the client that their progress is being actively monitored. It also provides an opportunity to regularly attend to their comfort, ensure that their dietary needs are met and their fluid intake is adequate, and determine if their medication requires adjustment.

Box 15.2 Guidelines for monitoring

- Two to four hourly observations, depending on severity of withdrawal symptoms.
- Orientate client to day, time and place.
- Check fluid balance. Offer fruit juices and avoid caffeinated beverages.
- Encourage a light diet if tolerated.
- Keep questions short, simple and avoid jargon.
- Avoid arguments with the client.
- Check level of comfort. Are extra blankets required? Does the client need showering?

Supportive care

Supportive care includes providing the client with:

- information
- reassurance
- an appropriate environment.

Information has been demonstrated to allay fear and anxiety in the withdrawal process.[9] The information given should include orientation to the setting and the staff, rules and regulations of the unit, the likely course of withdrawals and the medications which will be used, the blood tests that are likely to be ordered and introduction to the primary caregiver. Reassurance should be directed to allaying any fears about withdrawal symptoms, and positive feedback about progress. Where possible, information and reassurance should also be given to family members or concerned others. The environment in which detoxification occurs is very important. It should be calm, restful, quiet, uncluttered and non-threatening. Noisy visitors should be discouraged and any bright lights dimmed.

Pharmacotherapy

Pharmacotherapy is aimed at titrating the prescribed medication to the severity of withdrawal. While a number of medications have been used for this purpose, e.g. chlordiazepoxide (Librium), the current drug of choice

---

Box 15.3 Pharmacotherapy

Mild withdrawals:	5–10 mg of diazepam given every six to eight hours for two to four days.
Moderate to severe withdrawals:	diazepam administered on the first day as a loading dose of 20 mg, and if necessary every two hours to a total of 100 mg. Because of the long half-life of the drug this may be all that is required for the withdrawal episode. If not, 5–10 mg can be given every six hours for two to four days.
Severe withdrawals with hallucinations:	haloperidol (Serenace) is used as an adjunct therapy with diazepam. The dose is usually 2.5–5 mg repeated after one hour if required. It is seldom necessary to administer further doses.
Nausea or vomiting:	metoclopramide (Maxolon) 10 mg or prochlorperazine (Stemetil) 5 mg every four to six hours.
Diarrhoea:	Lomotil 5 mg two or three times a day as necessary, or Kaomagma 15–30 ml pro re nata.
Vitamin therapy:	problem drinkers should be considered to be vitamin deficient, and replacement is essential. The most important vitamin is thiamine (vitamin B_1), which is used to prevent the onset of Wernicke's encephalopathy. Thiamine should be given prophylactically, in doses of 100 mg two or three times a day for two weeks.

is diazepam.[5] This is because of the long half-life of the drug (18–40 hours) and its metabolites (two to five days). The drugs and doses used are generally the preferred choice of the prescribing doctor, and the regime provided in Box 15.3 is offered as a guide to what is becoming accepted as best practice.

Key point: Barbiturates and major tranquillisers should not be used routinely in the management of alcohol withdrawal, and oversedation should be avoided as it may mask underlying symptoms.[5]

Blood tests

The following tests are likely to be ordered: MCV red-cell count, liver function tests (GGT, ALP, ALT, AST), uric acid, lipids, hepatitis B surface antigen, hepatitis C and HIV antibody (if liver pathology is confirmed or illicit drug use suspected).[5]

Client perceptions of alcohol withdrawal

While the objective symptoms of the alcohol withdrawal syndrome are well documented, little attention has been given to how clients perceive the experience. The following is an extract from an interview with a client that illustrates how he felt during withdrawal in a specialist alcohol and drug unit:

> *'I was violently ill as soon as I arrived, vomiting and shaking and with diarrhoea. The nurses gave medication which they said I needed, and I was put to bed. I didn't sleep for two nights because I was scared my heart would stop beating. I thought I was going to stop breathing because my throat seemed to be closing up, and I had the shakes and hot and cold sweats. I didn't fit this time, but I have done so before and that is frightening. The nurses were very good. They were always there when I needed to talk and they helped me through it. Detox is a scary experience.'*

This client was a 32-year-old with a long history of heavy drinking. He had experienced three previous detoxifications, and had fitted during the last episode. His withdrawal symptoms had been treated with the pharmacotherapy described above, and he had required second-hourly monitoring and supportive care for two days. At no time had the scores on the CIWA-AR exceeded 15, and his severity of withdrawal was assessed as being moderate and uncomplicated. The above comments illustrate the anxiety felt by many clients undergoing withdrawals, and the importance of frequent contact, reassurance and supportive care during the process.

Key point: Supportive care and monitoring is the key to effective and efficient management of withdrawal symptoms.

Where should detoxification take place?

There is a growing body of evidence that the majority of individuals seeking withdrawal from alcohol do not require in-patient care. Out-patient management has been demonstrated to be effective for people with limited social supports,[10] with no severe medical or psychiatric complications,[11] and single, homeless people have been safely managed in a hostel.[12] Nor do all require sedation or specialist medical intervention. In a study of 1114 consecutive admissions to an alcohol detoxification unit, all but 90 were treated with vitamin therapy and supportive care.[13] In another study of approximately 5000 people who experienced withdrawal at St Vincent's Hospital, Sydney, only 51 required admission to a hospital and only one fatality occurred over several years of operation.[14]

Alcohol withdrawal can also be carried out in the home. Withdrawal at home has been demonstrated to be safe, acceptable to the person concerned and family, and is more cost-effective than in-patient care.[7,15,16]

Risk factors for home withdrawal

The risk factors that must be considered when assessing people for withdrawal in the home are related to the individual and the setting.

Individual

In addition to the factors itemised under Assessment, information should be obtained on the following:

- failure to complete previous home or out-patient-based withdrawal
- geographical and social isolation.

Setting

When assessing the suitability of the home as a setting for withdrawal, the Home Environment Assessment (HEA) is a useful tool.[7] On a range of 0–3 this scale allows a quantifiable assessment of the:

- availability of a support person
- attitude of the support person
- commitment of the support person
- presence of young children and or pets
- general atmosphere and level of noise in the home
- presence of other drinkers.

All these factors have a strong influence on how withdrawal will be experienced in the home. The maximum score on the scale is 24, and high scores indicate that the home setting is likely to be unsuitable for withdrawal. Comprehensive guidelines for home withdrawal have been produced.[7,17]

The advantages of withdrawal in the home are that the person is in familiar surroundings, partners or support persons are more readily able to be involved in the withdrawal process and choices about short- and long-term goals can be negotiated with all concerned. This is important as all members of a family are affected by problem drinking behaviour. It also avoids the stigma associated with being treated at designated alcohol agencies.

The disadvantages are that the home may contain cues to drinking. In other words, a lot of drinking may have taken place in the home and access to alcohol may be easy and undermine the person's resolve to abstain. It can also place an additional burden on a family that is already stressed. On the other hand, people undergoing withdrawal in the home avoid the 're-entry phase' experienced by those who have undergone withdrawal as an in-patient when they return to the environments from whence they came.

Case studies

The following case studies (1–3) serve to illustrate the importance of the home environment in home withdrawal. The first highlights the benefits of a supportive environment, the second the negative outcome of attempting withdrawal in an unsuitable setting.

CASE STUDY 1

John was a happily married, 35-year-old man with two young children. He owned a small contracting business, and he and his wife enjoyed a busy social life. John had been a regular, social drinker for many years without experiencing any problems related to alcohol.

During a time of economic depression, however, work became more competitive and eventually his contracting business was closed, and he was unable to find alternative employment. At this time his drinking increased to a point that his wife threatened to leave him if he did not get help.

John presented to a specialist alcohol and drug treatment agency, seeking withdrawal from alcohol. A comprehensive medical assessment indicated that he had no major physical or psychiatric conditions, and he was considered for home withdrawal. Pharmacotherapy was prescribed and a number of blood tests were performed. The home environment was assessed as suitable by a clinical nurse specialist (CNS). With the support and encouragement of his wife, John successfully completed withdrawal at home. The CNS visited daily for four days, his wife monitored the medication, nutrition and hygiene, and John was engaged in further counselling for his other problems. To what extent his economic position improved is unknown.

This is an example of a person in difficult financial circumstances undergoing a successful home withdrawal with the support of his family. Withdrawal did not solve the economic problems, but the family was in a better position to address them when John was sober.

CASE STUDY 2

James was a 28-year-old living in a *de facto* relationship in rented accommodation. He had a long history of heavy drinking and had recently lost his job. He was accepted for home withdrawal on the basis that he had no concurrent physical or psychiatric conditions, his partner was willing to be involved in the management and the home was assessed as suitable. On the second day, however, some friends visited with a supply of alcohol and James commenced drinking with them. When his partner objected, an argument ensued and she left the premises. A CNS reassessed the situation and the detoxification process was ceased. James was provided with telephone numbers of healthcare providers to contact if he wished to make another attempt to withdraw.

This is an example of an unsuccessful attempt to withdraw from alcohol in the home. Though the home was assessed as suitable, it was not possible to control the visitors or the effect that people drinking in the setting had on James' resolve to abstain from alcohol.

The majority of those presenting for alcohol withdrawal can be managed in the home or as an out-patient. Those who are likely to experience severe withdrawal symptoms or have a concurrent medical condition, however, should be managed as an in-patient in a hospital or specialist alcohol and drug unit with appropriate residential facilities.

Planned or unplanned

The above examples relate to when withdrawal has been planned. That is, when a person has contacted service providers for the purpose of undergoing detoxification. Withdrawal is often unplanned, and can occur in hospitals where it is not the main focus of care, but in which it may happen in concurrence with the condition for which the person concerned was admitted, for example when a person is admitted because of trauma or some sudden illness, and exhibits withdrawal symptoms because their accustomed level of alcohol consumption has been interrupted (case study 3).

CASE STUDY 3

Peter was a 40-year-old who had been drinking consistently on a daily basis for several years. He did not consider that he had been drinking excessively, and had no problems related to his alcohol use. He was involved in a car accident on his way home from work, sustained several fractures that required surgery and spent a week in hospital. The day after surgery he became anxious, agitated, somewhat disorientated and uncooperative. His pulse rate was increased and his blood pressure was elevated. His accustomed alcohol intake had not been noted on admission, and it was some time before his symptoms were diagnosed as withdrawal and brought under control.

If it had been possible to include a drinking history in his initial assessment, a care plan could have been devised to take into account the likelihood of withdrawal and the symptoms described above could have been avoided or ameliorated.

There are a number of options available for people wishing to undergo withdrawal from alcohol (Figure 15.1). For those who meet the criteria, the preferred option is the home, with support from the family and a visiting CNS and close liaison with the family's general practitioner. Other options could include in-patient management for perhaps two days, followed by daily monitoring as an out-patient. Another could be an overnight stay as

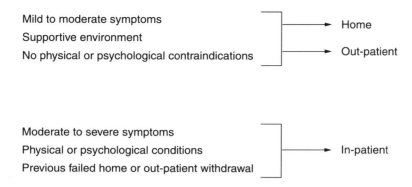

Mild to moderate symptoms — Home

Supportive environment

No physical or psychological contraindications — Out-patient

Moderate to severe symptoms

Physical or psychological conditions — In-patient

Previous failed home or out-patient withdrawal

Figure 15.1 Withdrawal settings.

an in-patient, followed up by home management. These options should be considered when assessing people for withdrawal, and are more flexible and responsive to individual needs than strict-adherence in-patient, out-patient or home-based care.

Conclusion

Most treatment programmes for individuals dependent on psychoactive drugs begin with detoxification. Detoxification programmes provide a humane way for individuals to undergo the withdrawal process and offer an opportunity for people to break the cycle of dependency on drugs. Following detoxification, it is important to offer clients a referral for follow-up care in the community. Detoxification, from any drug, is seldom sufficient to achieve long-term lifestyle changes, but it is a first step in the process.

To develop your knowledge in this area, see 'To learn more', p. 269.

Self-assessment questions

1 What are the signs and symptoms of the alcohol withdrawal syndrome?
2 Who is at risk of experiencing severe withdrawals?
3 What should a comprehensive client assessment include?
4 How would you monitor a client experiencing the alcohol withdrawal syndrome?
5 What are the risk factors for withdrawal in the home?

CHAPTER 16

Treatment and therapeutic interventions

Anne E Bartu

Pre-reading exercise

You have a client who has just completed detoxification. How would you determine what treatment would best assist the client to maintain this lifestyle change? What treatment or interventions would you suggest:

- for clients living in urban centres?
- for clients residing in rural areas?

When you have read the chapter, repeat the exercise to see if your understanding is the same or has improved. This exercise should take no more than 20 minutes to complete.

What constitutes treatment for alcohol dependence or alcohol-related problems? What constitutes a therapeutic intervention? Both terms are often used but rarely defined, and the distinction between them is blurred. Treatment and interventions are both aimed at changing a person's drinking behaviour. In addition they generally include activities designed to improve a person's health, psychological and social conditions as well as reducing their alcohol consumption. In many studies the term intervention is synonymous with treatment, or at times is used to refer to one or more components of a treatment modality. Interventions have been described as 'early', 'brief' or 'minimal'.[1] Early intervention involves detecting persons using alcohol or other drugs in a potentially hazardous manner and encouraging and assisting them to discontinue or moderate use before problems or dependence develop.[1] Early intervention is a form of case finding and treatment of early-stage problem drinkers. A brief or minimal intervention has been referred to as one that involves a minimum of expensive professional time.[2] Early intervention overlaps with brief intervention because both are relatively short in comparison with interventions that may be offered to people at a later stage in their drug-using career. It has been suggested, however, that the term 'early' is inappropriate as many people so designated will not progress to more serious problems.[3] Early and brief interventions have been recommended for use in generalist and primary healthcare settings for people who may be drinking at hazardous or harmful levels, but who may not be dependent on alcohol. They are not suitable for people dependent on alcohol.

Treatment is increasingly seen as a continuum that includes a range of activities, techniques or interventions that vary in content, duration, intensity, goals and settings, and are delivered by a number of healthcare workers from differing professional backgrounds such as doctors, nurses, psychologists, social workers and others.[3] Some forms of treatment that are used for people with alcohol problems are presented in Box 16.1.

Box 16.1 Forms of treatment

- Counselling
- Group therapy
- Aversion therapy
- Behavioural self-control
- Community reinforcement
- Family therapy
- Social skills training
- Pharmacotherapy
- Stress management
- Alcohol education
- Acupuncture
- Hypnosis
- Cue exposure

The list presented in Box 16.1 is not in order of priority, nor is it all-inclusive. It serves to illustrate some of the interventions or treatments that have been, and are being, used to assist people with drinking problems. Viewed as such they represent a smorgasbord of techniques that are not appropriate for all clients, and are not uniformly available in all areas. One way of viewing treatment for alcohol-dependent people is to consider it occurring in a series of stages in which a number of activities or interventions relevant to that stage are provided for the client (Box 16.2).

> **Box 16.2** Stages of treatment
>
> Stage 1   Detoxification
> Stage 2   Rehabilitation/follow-up
> Stage 3   Maintenance

Stage One

The first stage is detoxification. As discussed in Chapter 15, detoxification is the management of the withdrawal symptoms that occur when a person dependent on alcohol ceases drinking. Detoxification can be planned or unplanned, and can take place in a number of settings. Detoxification alone is seldom sufficient to maintain any long-term lifestyle change. It is only part of the process, and many adjustments are necessary to maintain short or long-term goals. Further treatment or interventions are required to assist the client during this period following detoxification.

Stage Two

Stage two is rehabilitation. This can be experienced in a residential facility, or more commonly on an out-patient basis at a treatment agency. Following detoxification, a comprehensive assessment of the individual's physical, social and psychological status and environmental factors that may have contributed to their drinking problem is conducted. The assessment may indicate that the person needs new coping or other skills to prevent relapse to drinking. Skills training can be used to address any deficits that may have led to drinking as a coping strategy. The skills recommended as useful are assertiveness, drink refusal, social skills, relaxation, stress management and relationship enhancement.[1]

One of the most important issues for people dependent on alcohol who are attempting to change their drinking behaviour is relapse prevention. A number of pharmacotherapeutic agents such as bromocriptine, buspirone, disulfiram, naltrexone and acamprosate have been used to assist people to maintain abstinence. The list is not all-inclusive. While disulfiram has possibly been used most frequently for this purpose, acamprosate is the first drug specifically designed to maintain abstinence post-detoxification in alcohol-dependent clients. None of these drugs should be considered if the person's goal is controlled drinking.

Disulfiram

Disulfiram, or Antabuse, is an alcohol-sensitising agent that inhibits the action of the enzyme aldehyde dehydrogenase. This causes a disulfiram ethanol reaction (DER) that is manifested in nausea, flushing, diarrhoea, breathing problems, peripheral neuritis and fluctuating blood pressure. Disulfiram may also, in rare cases, induce toxic hepatitis, but according to Brewer,[4] the toxicity of the drug has been overstated. Adverse effects can appear within 20 minutes of drinking and, though transient, can last up to 90–180 minutes. The symptoms of DER can also be experienced two to three days after the person concerned has ceased to take the drug if they have returned to drinking.

Dosage
The prescribed dose of disulfiram is usually 200–250 mg taken orally, daily, for three to six months.[5] An alternative mode of administration is by surgical implant in subcutaneous tissue, however there is no consensus on the benefits of this over the oral mode. Disulfiram should not be commenced unless the patient has been abstinent from alcohol for 24 hours.[5]

Disulfiram is not recommended for routine use for all people dependent on alcohol. People should not take disulfiram if:

• they are pregnant
• they have any concurrent medical or psychiatric problems.

The efficacy of disulfiram is said to be increased when the person taking the medication is in a stable relationship, and the daily dose is able to be supervised.[5]

Acamprosate

Acamprosate is a synthetic compound, similar to gamma-aminobutyric acid (GABA), thought to inhibit multiple neurotransmitter systems, reduce craving and reduce alcohol consumption.[6] The adverse effects may include diarrhoea, and less commonly nausea and vomiting may occur. In a review of the pharmacology and clinical potential of acamprosate in the management of alcohol dependence after detoxification, Wilde and Wagstaff concluded that, as an adjunct to psychosocial and behavioural interventions, acamprosate offers a promising advance in maintaining post-detoxification abstinence.[6] They qualify this, however, by stating that more studies are required to confirm the favourable outcomes reported.

Dosage

It is suggested that acamprosate should be initiated immediately following the withdrawal period and treatment maintained for one year. The recommended dose is 1.3 g/day for patients weighing <60 kg and 2 g/day for patients weighing >60 kg, given daily in divided doses for up to one year. Acamprosate is contraindicated for pregnant or lactating women, patients with renal or hepatic impairment, or the elderly.[6]

Stage Three

The third phase is maintenance. This refers to ongoing support for a person after they have completed a formal treatment programme. It can be provided in the form of informal contact with the treatment agency or by participation in self-help groups. Possibly the best known of the self-help groups is Alcoholics Anonymous (AA). AA functions on the premise that alcoholism is a disease which cannot be cured but can be arrested through abstinence. A more experienced AA member sponsors those attending AA groups or offered social support, and helps them work through what are called the '12 steps of recovery'. The 12 steps include admitting that they have no control over alcohol, and placing their recovery in the hands of a higher power. They also subject themselves to critical self-examination, make a commitment to honesty and humility, and accept the reality of the past, the harm they have caused and responsibility for restitution of harm done. Frequent attendance at meetings is recommended, and members are welcomed back time and again should they relapse to drinking.[7]

Other programmes based on the 12 steps are Al-Anon and Al-Teen. Al-Anon is designed to help family members deal with the problems generated by having a problem drinker in the family. Al-Teen is designed for teenagers who have an alcohol-dependent parent or parents. As the goal is abstinence, AA is not suitable for anyone who is seeking to continue drinking, albeit in a reduced or controlled manner. The self-help groups of AA are highly accessible and offer clients social support from others who have had similar experiences with alcohol. In some areas AA may be the only source of support available. Attendance at AA groups is not confined to stage three. In many treatment facilities people are introduced to AA in stage one, and the 12 steps form the basis for many rehabilitation programmes.

How long are the stages of treatment?

The time spent in each stage depends on a person's level of dependency (both physical and psychological), motivation to change and social and environmental factors. In general, however:

- detoxification takes from three to four days
- rehabilitation takes from six to 12 months
- maintenance may be lifelong.

The stages are not clearly bounded. For example, some withdrawal symptoms such as sleep disturbances may continue to be experienced well into the rehabilitation stage, and apart from formal separation from a rehabilitation treatment programme it is difficult to determine when maintenance commences. The interventions mentioned above are also not confined to specific stages, for example counselling occurs in stage one and two, and possibly in stage three. Alcohol education is frequently provided in stage one and is reinforced in stage two. Group therapy is often provided in stage one, and in some form or another continues in the other stages, and assessment is ongoing in all stages. In addition, not all clients will consent to protracted rehabilitation programmes, and many will opt for ongoing support following detoxification from AA alone.

Counselling

No one would deny that counselling has an important role in treatment. While counselling alone is seldom enough to bring about change in drinking behaviours, the use of good counselling skills assists in building a trusting relationship with clients. The approach to counselling is that proposed by Egan.[8] This is based on empathy, the use of open-ended questions, reflective listening, affirmations and summarising. The use of confrontational techniques is avoided. According to Egan, the most important counselling skill is empathy. Empathy involves listening to clients in a non-judgemental manner, and attempting to understand problems and issues from their perspective. It includes helping clients to find solutions to their problems rather than offering solutions to them. In this approach the responsibility for change lies with the client, not the counsellor.

For the alcohol and drug field it has been suggested that the above approach to counselling would be enhanced if it was combined with motivational interviewing (*see also* Chapter 13).[1] The main components of motivational interviewing are empathy, highlighting discrepancies between behaviour and goals, avoiding confrontation and arguments with the client, 'rolling' with the client's resistance to change and supporting the client's belief in their ability to change.[9]

Linking to services

The challenge in developing treatment plans for clients following detoxification is to link or match them with appropriate interventions. To receive optimal treatment, clients should be matched to interventions that address their specific problems and lifestyles.[10] This implies that certain treatments would be better for certain types of clients. Recently, a large national, multisite, randomised clinical trial of alcoholism treatment matching, entitled *Matching Alcoholism Treatments to Client Heterogeneity* (Project MATCH), was completed in the United States of America.[11] The aims of the project were to assess the benefits of matching alcohol-dependent clients to three different treatments with reference to a variety of client outcomes. The three treatments were (1) cognitive behavioural coping skills therapy, (2) motivational enhancement therapy and (3) 12-step facilitation therapy. Two independent clinical trials were conducted, one with alcohol-dependent clients receiving out-patient therapy, and one with clients receiving aftercare therapy following in-patient or day hospital treatment. Clients were monitored over a one-year post-treatment period and evaluated on a number of matching variables.

The primary outcome measures were percentage of days abstinent and drinks per drinking day. The results indicated that only psychiatric severity demonstrated a significant treatment interaction, and no single treatment showed an overall superiority in terms of post-treatment success, regardless of what outcome measure was employed. Despite these findings it is sound clinical practice to devise, in conjunction with the client, strategies and interventions to assist them to achieve their goals. This requires:

• a comprehensive assessment of the client and their social environment
• sound knowledge of the services available.

This includes knowledge of appropriate agencies and self-help groups, up-to-date information on their location, services or programmes, and whether or not they actually deliver what they advertise. Services for people with alcohol and other drug problems are not distributed equitably. Few areas have a full complement of services, and some are almost totally deficient. While it is possible to determine what would best meet a client's needs through a comprehensive assessment, the reality is that attempts to link clients with appropriate services are limited by availability. In many cases, this is less than optimal.

Case studies

The following case studies serve to illustrate the importance of the availability of services for clients following detoxification. The first highlights the benefits of availability of a full range of follow-up or rehabilitation services, the second the problems faced by individuals when no services are available.

CASE STUDY 1

Margaret was a 28-year-old woman, married with three young children. She lived in an urban area and worked part-time in a florist shop. Following a successful in-patient detoxification, it was determined that she would benefit from some training in relaxation, stress management and coping. Her long-term drinking goal was controlled drinking. Though there was a residential rehabilitation agency in the vicinity, it was deemed unsuitable because it was abstinent oriented and, moreover, Margaret needed to be home to care for her children. Margaret had follow-up care on an out-patient basis at the agency in which she had experienced detoxification. She attended three times a week for three months, addressed her skills deficits in group therapy and commenced a controlled drinking programme.

This is an example of linking a person to appropriate and available follow-up services that enabled her to improve her life skills, work towards her drinking goals and maintain her family obligations.

CASE STUDY 2

David was a 38-year-old man who lived in a rural area. He was married with two children and was self-employed. Following detoxification his assessment indicated that he would benefit from stress-management training and family therapy. His drinking goal was abstinence. Unfortunately there were no services in his area to provide the follow-up he required, and he could not leave his business to seek them elsewhere in a rehabilitation agency. He was linked to the local chapter of AA and attended meetings twice a week. While he would gain a considerable amount of support from the group, training in stress management and family therapy were unavailable.

This is an example of the reality for many people. While assessments may indicate that certain interventions or training are required to support a person in the follow-up stage, in many cases a review of their geographical availability highlights the deficiencies in distribution.

Conclusion

Treatment has come to be viewed as a continuum that includes a variety of interventions that may be provided for clients according to need and availability. Both interventions and treatment have the same goals, that is, to assist individuals to reduce the harms associated with alcohol misuse. Rather than seeking to distinguish between the two terms, it is more useful to consider treatment occurring in a series of stages in which a number of interventions may be provided. Inherent to all treatment is counselling: the approach recommended is the non-confrontational technique proposed by Egan,[8] linked with motivational interviewing. The assessment of clients for rehabilitation and maintenance should include a review of the person's resources and needs and an overview of what is available to meet these needs. While this will indicate what is required, it will also highlight any deficiencies in the distribution of the location of services. Despite the gains made in treatment for people with alcohol problems over the last decade, unless they are accessible to those in need the options are limited to what is available.

To develop your knowledge in this area, see 'To learn more', p. 270.

Self-assessment questions

1 How should treatment be viewed?
2 What are the main stages of treatment?
3 What counselling approach should be used?
4 What should a comprehensive assessment include?
5 What are the limiting factors in linking clients to optimal services?

CHAPTER 17

Creating common ground

Susan A Storti and Olga Maranjian Church

Pre-reading exercise

There are any number of good reasons to engage in the process of interdisciplinary team building. The umbrella under which most reasons fall includes the belief that effective teams enable an organisation to accomplish its goals and objectives in a timely and effective manner.

Following are 10 questions. Please respond by circling the number corresponding to your experience: 1 = least applicable, 5 = most applicable **or** 1 = strongly disagree, 5 = strongly agree.

Teams are an effective way of treating substance abuse.	1 2 3 4 5
Teams are an efficient way of treating substance abuse.	1 2 3 4 5
Teams can work for everyone.	1 2 3 4 5
Teams are of benefit to the client.	1 2 3 4 5
Group trust builds because individual team members come through on their commitments.	1 2 3 4 5
There is an absence of competition between team members.	1 2 3 4 5
Non-judgemental accurately describes the attitude toward the differences present within a team.	1 2 3 4 5
I believe I can effectively work with an interdisciplinary team.	1 2 3 4 5
I understand what is required to make a team work.	1 2 3 4 5
I want to work with an interdisciplinary team.	1 2 3 4 5

Introduction

In the United States, 'the healthcare system is evolving in unprecedented ways. Individually based practices are giving way to multi-group and managed-care systems. Hospitals are merging into larger systems that offer out-patient facilities as well as preventive social and ancillary services'.[1]

Interdisciplinary pursuits are being encouraged in order to meet healthcare needs of communities as well as clients. Since many disciplines contribute to the delivery of healthcare it seems obvious that meaningful progress in providing better healthcare cannot be accomplished by one discipline working in isolation. At the same time, experts point to a 'worrisome gap' between client needs and the actual provision of competent skill-based care, while changes in the workplace demand that the workforce provides higher quality at lower costs.

Although the current rhetoric speaks to working in interdisciplinary teams as a core skill for healthcare professionals, the change towards such teamwork is at best slow. Nowhere is this more true than in behavioural healthcare and, in particular, in the field of addictions. For the purpose of this chapter, behavioural healthcare is defined as the term used in today's managed-care environment and as a phrase that encompasses preventive and treatment programmes in mental health and mental illness, including addictions.

In general, health professions' education still focuses on the one-to-one method of care. Research findings[2] reveal that almost 40% of physicians felt inadequately prepared for work in healthcare teams. The deficit for all healthcare professionals is a profound lack of preparation and or opportunities to experience the knowledge, skills and valuable outcomes that come from effective teamwork. As reported by McEwen,[3] 'The Pew commission supports revision of curricula to include "healthcare teamwork" in which the educational and care delivery arrangements of schools should model the integration of healthcare providers'.

The challenge for educators and practitioners in the behavioural healthcare field is to be aware of this deficit and become actively involved in identifying and developing collaborative opportunities for both didactic and experiential learning. Understanding the parameters of our practice ultimately will lead to a greater chance for a comprehensive, collaborative approach to the delivery of quality care. For example, often although individuals from various disciplines working with substance-abusing clients might have the same ultimate goal, i.e. change in drinking behaviour, the messages conveyed individually may be fragmented, disconnected and even counterproductive. In addition, the client may seek to sustain such disconnected care, playing one against the other in the interest of maintaining distance from reaching the goal of change.

The problems and possibilities are multidimensional and the pervasive nature of substance use in most societies, as well as the United States, requires a rapid reorientation to the ways in which we teach and learn. One opportunity to integrate a variety of perspectives and approaches to substance-using clients and their care was provided by a federally funded project, The Addiction Technology Transfer Center of New England (ATTC-NE). The interdisciplinary task force of the ATTC-NE developed introductory instructional modules for team building in the interest of providing effective higher quality and lower cost care to substance-using clients.

The Addiction Technology Transfer Center of New England was initiated in 1993 in response to a perceived shortage in the public sector of well-trained addiction treatment professionals. The ATTC-NE, located at Brown University's Center for Alcohol and Addiction Studies, is a consortium of state governors and university representatives from the six New England states – Vermont, Maine, Massachusetts, New Hampshire, Connecticut and Rhode Island. Recognising the rapid and dramatic changes occurring in the organisation and delivery of addictions and other health services, the ATTC-NE endorsed a collaborative approach among various disciplines.

The interdisciplinary initiative

Within the ATTC-NE, a task force – composed of nurses, physicians, social workers and counsellors – came together to discuss issues and concerns that impact on the development of interdisciplinary education in alcohol, tobacco and other drug abuse (ATODA).

In developing our curriculum modules, 'interdisciplinary' was defined as:

> '*a group of people, each of whom possesses particular expertise; each of whom is responsible for making individual decisions; who together hold common purposes and who meet together to communicate, collaborate and consolidate knowledge.*'[4]

The term 'discipline' signifies tools, methods, procedures, concepts and theories that account coherently for a set of objects or concepts. Over time they are shaped and reshaped by external contingencies and internal intellectual demands. In this manner a discipline comes to organise and concentrate experience into a particular 'world view'.[5] This world view not only defines but also limits the methods, concepts, questions, answers and criteria for truth and validity – in short, the particular parameters of a given discipline's image of reality. As Burke[6] states, 'A way of seeing is also a way of not seeing!'.

In order to develop an entity beyond each discipline, our explorations transcended discipline-specific boundaries. This entity, for lack of a better name, is the team, and what we explored was teamwork. For we believed good interdisciplinary care is based on good teamwork – and both are based on excellent communications skills, and good interdisciplinary education and training.

It was also important to clarify the levels of interdisciplinary interactions. By gathering several different disciplines together without true interaction, with each member bringing and holding their own world view, no wider vision would be created – we simply would have a multidisciplinary meeting, i.e. a group representing many disciplines.

We determined that interdisciplinary interactions are those in which different disciplines support solutions and create *common ground* by transcending their discipline-specific boundaries.

Social work researchers[7] studying conflict in interdisciplinary team life concluded that, in general, team members see themselves as representative of their discipline rather than members of a whole that transcends individual disciplines. Perspectives are splintered rather than united. Team members may want to come to consensus but there are barriers to integrating their findings. The literature suggests that there is a hierarchy of disciplines as well as external factors that influence team processes. In addition to such status issues there are other barriers to effective collaboration.

Barriers across disciplines were identified as follows:

- lack of understanding of other disciplines' roles and responsibilities (i.e. lack of awareness of contributions from others)
- increased anxiety regarding roles and responsibilities (i.e. boundary anxiety due to managed care initiatives, funding, economic considerations and competition around overlap and gaps)
- wide variance in work roles and responsibilities, diversity of setting and administration related to:
  - semantic problems as well as differing language
  - discipline disempowerment when not represented in the chosen method of treatment (MOT)
  - initial time-consuming coordination for interdisciplinary integration which results in increased economic output
  - inconsistency in treatment approaches
  - conceptual models and organising framework for approaching the problem.

In addition we identified the following potential barriers basic *to each of our disciplines*:

- lack of overall recognition of ATODA within each of our educational programmes
- lack of standardisation in ATODA skills for each discipline
- lack of role models for the ATODA role in each discipline
- overall discipline-specific task orientation
- frequent rotation of assignments within training and education programmes disruptive to developing and maintaining interactions across disciplines.

What became increasingly obvious was that each discipline has its own 'culture'. With this in mind, an anthropologist was consulted to assist us as we dealt with our 'cultural' differences. As a result, insights and new directions led us to the following goals:

- to promote collaboration among ATODA educators, practitioners and researchers
- to promote understanding of similarities and differences in the roles and responsibilities of individual disciplines within the ATODA 'team'
- to identify possibilities and potential for comparative collaborative inter-disciplinary education and research
- to provide an ongoing forum for discussion and the development, im-plementation and evaluation of an interdisciplinary model or learning modules for ATODA education and practice.

As we approached our task we found that we needed to clarify relative responsibilities to ensure effective, efficient and appropriate responses to the needs of people we serve. Our initial meetings were spent in developing a matrix, which graphically identified roles and responsibilities and functions of all four disciplines involved. Both the micro approach, i.e. distinguishing disciplines, and the macro approach, i.e. identifying universal elements, were all parts of the puzzle.

By developing this matrix first, we sought a coherent, convergent model that visually revealed the similarities and differences, i.e. the areas of overlap as well as the gaps in our various approaches to our clients. It has been said that 'a group becomes a team when all members are sure enough of themselves and their contributions to praise the skill of others' (Anonymous). This is perhaps the most important finding from our initiative. Each member of each discipline must feel they can safely share, and trust that their professional boundaries will not be eroded.

The paradox of a true interdisciplinary approach is that it relies on the competence and mastery of discipline-specific knowledge, expertise and accountability, as well as a willingness to share, in the development of common ground.

The challenge continues – piloting and reviewing the curriculum

Prior to piloting the project, the curriculum was forwarded to individuals at federal, national, regional and state level who are considered experts in substance use and its related issues, for content review. These included individuals from various ethnic and minority groups, as well as the disciplines of social work, nursing, medicine, psychology, and counselling, administrators, researchers, managed care contractors, the academic faculty, private training contractors and clinical supervisors. They were geographically situated across the United States and Puerto Rico. Of the 32 copies forwarded for review, we received feedback from 25 of the identified experts. We asked them to review the curriculum for content, format, applicability and accuracy.

Upon receipt of the feedback, we incorporated the comments and recommendations into the existing curriculum. We then proceeded to send a letter of invitation to each of the six New England Single State Drug and Alcohol Agencies, offering them an opportunity to collaborate with the ATTC-NE in piloting this curriculum. It was described as an introductory, instructional curriculum, designed as a two-day training course to educate professionals from different disciplines to work through the group dynamic of team building. We requested that two to three individuals from each agency who were representative of different disciplines be invited to participate. We also requested that the agencies invited to attend should be in the planning stages of team development or have an interest in developing interdisciplinary teams for the delivery of substance-use services.

Seventeen individuals became involved, representing five agencies: one substance use treatment agency and four substance use and mental health agencies. Each group had representation from nursing, social work, counselling and, in one group, administration. The participants felt that these groupings were representative of what actually occurred in the clinical setting.

All participants completed the programme. During the course of the two-day training, the groups were asked to participate in several activities simulating team development. The exercises ranged from developing a mission statement for the team to developing an action plan for specific agencies. For example, one such activity included reading a case study, discussing with team members and developing a treatment plan to meet the specific needs of the client described. During this process, several issues arose. First and foremost, the team had difficulty deciding what the primary diagnosis was: substance abuse or mental health. Second, as the treatment plan was being developed, territorial markings of each discipline became very apparent. Heated discussions ensued around each other's roles and responsibilities with respect to their specific discipline. This held especially true between the counsellors and caseworkers and the social workers. With some facilitation on the part of the instructors, these concerns were addressed and processed with all participants. Although the training did not provide the opportunity to experience the entire team-building process, it did provide an opportunity for experiential learning as well as the development or enhancement of communication skills among its participants.

Another such example occurred during the discussion about who would serve best in the role of leader and who in the role of facilitator. Here, the nurses present in the training immediately assumed that they should take a leadership position within the team, based solely on the fact that they felt that this was a 'natural' for them. The social workers were very quick to point out that they were as qualified and well versed as nurses, based on their academic preparation, and therefore they should assume the leader's role. This type of debate was deliberate on the part of the curriculum as it created an opportunity for the team members to talk to each other about their education and life experience, their present role within their agency and their responsibilities as part of their role. Participants quickly came to the realisation that although they may have been employed at the same agency, they did not have a full understanding of what each other did. They also found duplication within their work.

Whatever the case scenario presented, there was one area upon which all participants agreed. Although physicians were absent, the general consensus was that had physicians been present, they would have assumed the role of the leader. The instructors processed this with participants, asking questions such as: 'Why do you think physicians automatically assume this role?', 'Is it because we as healthcare providers see them in this role, or is it because this is how it is assumed to be?' and 'Were you, in each of your respective disciplines, taught that this is how it was to be when employed in a clinical setting?'

We then asked participants if any had worked in a team environment before and, if so, to provide a description of their experience. The participants were very happy to share their backgrounds, experiences and their perceptions and misconceptions about the roles and responsibilities of other disciplines.

In addition, questions relating to the utilisation of this model and the benefit of the training from a discipline-specific perspective were asked. Responses varied. For example, most agreed the content of each area reflected the overall objectives of the training. However, some felt that the content could be condensed, and although the training modules provided a general orientation to interdisciplinary team building, the need for adaptation to agency-specific services was evident.

A good example of adaptation of the basic concepts of this model involves the Rhode Island Municipal Police Training Academy (RIMPTA). In collaboration with the ATTC-NE, RIMPTA has tailored the curriculum and currently uses it as a foundation course for the development of community policing initiatives.

Following the training, the participants were asked to answer the same questions posed to our content reviewers, as well as some additional questions about applicability in a clinical setting from their discipline-specific perspective.

Advantages of interdisciplinary education and service

So, what are the advantages of working together? The advantages of teamwork as it relates to interdisciplinary education and service are as follows:

- multiple viewpoints from a variety of backgrounds
- increased resources
- shared workload
- increased skills and abilities for complex projects and problems
- opportunity for novices to develop
- opportunity to broaden personal networks
- answers wider variety of questions
- rewards of successful mutual endeavour.

Although our experience has been positive, we realise that we need to convince the policy makers and agency administrators that the concept of interdisciplinary teams is beneficial to the client and the agency in the delivery of treatment services. We need to stress the effectiveness of this approach, utilising outcome data for the populations we treat.

According to Katzenbach and Smith,[8] 'Teams outperform individuals acting alone or in larger organisational groupings, especially when performance requires multiple skills, judgements and experiences. Most people recognise the capabilities of teams: most have the common sense to make teams work. Nevertheless most people overlook team opportunities for themselves'.

The ATTC-NE interdisciplinary initiative is one step in the direction of assisting individuals within a variety of disciplines to identify and deal with the challenges and opportunities that may lead them toward true teamwork.

The attempt to create common ground in the midst of the current upheaval within the healthcare arena has contributed to a panoramic view of possibilities for the future. In today's context of change, it may be helpful to view '… the healthcare system as … a colossal jigsaw puzzle in which the parts – financing, organisation, service, training and people – are aligning themselves into a new order and a new fit'.[9] As the puzzle takes shape, we can expect that '… the quality of that picture depends on a joint capacity to assemble the pieces …'.

To develop your knowledge in this area, see 'To learn more', p. 270.

Self-assessment questions

Return to the assessment you completed prior to reading this chapter. Reflect on each of your responses. Based on your readings, would you answer any of them of differently? If yes, why?

Now attempt to answer the following questions:

1 Interdisciplinary interactions are those in which different disciplines support solutions, however maintaining their discipline-specific boundaries. True or false?
2 When does a group actually become a team?
3 To ensure effective, efficient and appropriate responses to patient needs, team members must have clarity about their relative role and responsibilities. True or false?
4 What is meant by a 'true interdisciplinary approach'?
5 What are some advantages of interdisciplinary education and service delivery?

CHAPTER 18

The need for *professional* communication

David B Cooper

Pre-reading exercise

Read the following questions before reading this chapter. When you have read the chapter repeat the second question to see if you could implement any changes that will improve the problems you identified in question 1.

1 When was the last time you wished communication within or outwith your team would improve? Now take a few moments to identify the problems.
2 What steps do you think *you* could have taken to improve the communication problems?

Introduction

This chapter specifically builds upon Chapter 17, 'Creating common ground', which looked at multidisciplinary teamwork. It is deliberately a general chapter related to individual practice and improving communication, something that is part of the daily life of each professional. It highlights the importance of communication in the identification, care, and in meeting the needs of the individuals we come into contact with on a daily basis.

This chapter will not be laden with references. It merely puts into perspective and provides a rationale for the common courtesy and practice that is part of the professional's daily activities. We become so familiar with such communication that it is easy to oversimplify its importance and consequently miss the considerable value it holds for individuals and groups alike.

'Communicate' is defined as 'To impart (knowledge) or exchange (thoughts) by speech, writing, gesture, etc. To have sympathetic mutual understanding'.[1] 'Communication' is defined as 'The imparting or exchange of information, ideas, feelings. Something communicated, such as a message'.[1] The strength of any local or national body lies in its ability to communicate effectively. Poor communication has a negative, knock-on effect on the care of the individual participating in the therapeutic intervention. Good working practices and relationships, working towards the identification of alcohol-related problems, can only be achieved locally and nationally if each professional takes responsibility to communicate effectively with the other. The professional can have an effective voice in policy development and the way service provision develops to meet the needs of the individual experiencing alcohol-related problems.

However, there are many good ideas and developments at local and national level that are never shared. The concept of keeping things within the organisation or professional group still exists. Often this stems from fears associated with funding. One organisation went as far as to ban members of staff giving information to clients or other organisations about the national drink helpline in case their local health authority cut funding to the service. Another organisation, developing a new approach to alcohol-related problems, refused to share this information because it was their idea! If we look at the concept of evidence-based practice within the realms of clinical governance, then we have a duty to disseminate knowledge and best practice in order to promote clinical excellence and effectiveness. If we do not communicate what it is we are doing, good or bad, at local and national level, how can we hope to identify and meet the needs of the individual experiencing alcohol-related problems, or encourage others that such identification is important to the consequences of the individual's health, and professional's own workload?

Many organisations have professional conduct rules, e.g. the United Kingdom Central Council for Nursing, Midwifery and Health Visiting (UKCC) lays clear obligations on the nurse as to his or her responsibilities to the patient or client:

> *'The only appropriate professional relationship between a client and a practitioner is one which focuses exclusively upon the needs of the client.'*[2]

> *'Registered nurses, midwives and health visitors must treat the client and the client's decisions about their own needs with respect. This involves identifying the client's own preferences regarding nursing, midwifery and health visiting care and respecting them within the limits of current standards of practice, existing legislation and the goals of the therapeutic relationship. Practitioners are personally accountable for ensuring that they promote and protect the interests of clients in their care, irrespective of gender, age, race, disability, sexuality, culture or religious beliefs.'*[3]

To do this effectively, we have to be able to offer the individual presenting for care the opportunity to examine their alcohol use, and communicate effectively with them and other health, spiritual and social care professionals.

Effective communication

The impact of verbal communication between professionals cannot be overemphasised. 'Communication is the master key. It fits all locks and opens all doors.'[4] How professionals share important and routine information related to the care of the individual, and those significant others within the individual's environment, can, and does, have a major impact on the successful outcome of any therapeutic intervention.

The health professional's life is hectic and full of twists, turns and manoeuvres. Consequently, it is easy to become enclosed within what we have to do, that is, the tasks of daily work, and to forget to inform other professionals and organisations involved in an individual's care of matters that impinge on their daily life. If this is left unmanaged, then communication breaks down and ill feeling and rivalry can ensue. When one is busy, time is of great importance, and visiting the client at home, for example, only to find the visit has clashed with an unknown out-patient or other appointment can leave the professional feeling frustrated and angry, as if time has been stolen.

Other examples include:

* the reserved hospital bed left unoccupied because the ward has not been informed of the patient or client's admission to another ward for other health reasons
* the wasted general practitioner appointment, or home visit, because no one has informed the surgery that the patient or client has been admitted to the hospital ward. Before there are cries of 'but the family should do that', any hospital admission, planned or unplanned, causes disruption and anxiety within a family. Even the most routine of admissions can cause fear, confusion and apprehension. At such times the family's main concern is for the patient, not the NHS! A simple enquiry as to whether the patient is due to see any other professional will elicit the information on which the relative can be advised to act, or upon which the professional can act
* the patient or client who is discharged home without notification of other professionals involved. Continuity of care is important at all times.

The above examples occur regularly. No one profession is to blame. Human nature dictates that we all look for short cuts to reduce the perceived workload without consideration of the 'knock-on' effect on others. The consequences of poor communication come from, and affect, all professional groups, thus affecting those who are receiving therapeutic interventions.

Of course, one can communicate with a colleague and still come across misunderstanding. Anyone who has a teenage son or daughter will know that even when the benefits of having a clean and tidy room have been explained for the hundredth time, a check has been made to ensure understanding, numerous reminders have been administered and consequences explained, the room remains uncleaned. We can only try to improve communication and to make this as clear and unambiguous as possible. Human nature dictates that some communications will go unheeded or misinterpreted.

At times of pressure and stress, effective communication is the first to suffer. Yet, effective communication actually reduces pressure and stress as it frees up time to deal with other matters important to patient or client care.

Effective communication comes from the top. If senior managers lead by example then employees find the tasks they are set easier to work with and control. However, a lack of such leadership is not an excuse for our own actions, inactions or omissions. So what forms can effective communication take? What can the individual professional do to improve personal communication with colleagues?

The following is designed to improve communication. In essence, common sense, courtesy and good manners form the basis of good communication so consider the following as a stepping stone. Allow for a lot of personal effort, patience and practice, and disappointment, but do keep trying the three 'Rs'– **R**epetition, **R**epetition, **R**epetition – as it is the key to success. It is possible to improve communication as an individual and as a team.

Communicating with a colleague

It is frustrating to feel that your professional communications within and outwith the team, at senior or subordinate levels, are not being heard and acted upon. It is essential to remember that communication is a two-way process. Often information needs reinforcement and clarification. Both parties need to understand what is required, what is said and, just as important, what is not said to keep the interaction and knock-on effect on patient or client intervention running smoothly. Do write, do telephone and do remember to thank people for their actions on your behalf. This is basic good manners, but often forgotten.

Communicating information

All care professionals receive copious amounts of written communication. It is easy to leave information in the in-tray until 'we have more time to deal with it'. Your own personal experience will tell you that such a time never arrives. It is essential to set regular time aside each day to deal with incoming and outgoing mail. If a communication is going to take time to deal with, telephone, e-mail or fax the originator of the communication to let them know when a reply to the communication can be expected. Add the date in your diary so that it can be checked and actioned later.

Some individuals within teams withhold information. To possess information that is not yet available to others is often misinterpreted as 'power'. Practice and service provision can only be improved effectively if information is shared. There is more 'power' and 'respect' from sharing information and resources with colleagues than from withholding it. After all, if no one knows you are holding that information, perhaps on a new treatment method or approach, how can your influence and knowledge over your colleagues be acknowledged! More importantly, how can *they* improve patient or client care!

One way to share information and ensure that it has been read is to circulate the document with a 'circulation list'. Each recipient signs the list to acknowledge receipt and to confirm it has been read. To be more effective, individual copies could be distributed.

Regular staff meetings are also essential in lubricating the sharing of information. If you are a 'hoarder' by nature, this will be your opportunity to demonstrate your skill and knowledge and at the same time bring the rest of the team up to date.

Communicating change

Change in any organisation is unsettling. Half-truths and rumours need little encouragement in dissemination and cause dissatisfaction. It is easier to have all your colleagues on board the ship than to stop the ship, circle and collect those who have fallen overboard (even if the ship is the *Titanic*!). Change affects all members of the team. To share and be fully conversant with the change and the process it takes can, and does, lead to team support. Involvement and a sense of being part of the change process rather than feeling excluded and unworthy of consideration is essential in effective communication and ownership of the change.

The admission process

In whichever area of health, spiritual, legal or social care you work, the admission or acceptance of a planned therapeutic interaction with a patient or client and or relative will be part of your role. To be effective it is essential we communicate with any significant others involved in the care of that individual. The primary worker needs to become the communication coordinator. However, this does not detract from the importance of all professionals being involved in ensuring that communications relating to that individual are effectively dealt with, otherwise, for example, in the case of emergency hospital admission, often the general practitioner, community nurse, social worker, occupational therapist, community psychiatric nurse or whoever is actively involved in the care is unaware that the admission has taken place. As soon as the individual is engaged with the professional, information should be gathered as to other services involved in the care, directly or indirectly. Planned appointments that may be missed or proposed community visits and or out-patient or client appointments need to be noted, and each professional colleague or agency informed.

With the patient's permission, information on their past and present health, spiritual or social problems can be discussed with each agency and a primary worker appointed. Just as important is the information available from the relative(s) (with the patient's permission). Often the patient or client can forget or feel unable to express important facts and information relevant to the presenting problem.

It is often easier to share information with other professionals using a multi-copy letter. It is good practice (and will be much appreciated by other colleagues) to give the patient or client a copy of this letter.

The discharge process

If the care needs of the patient or client have changed since your therapeutic intervention, it may be appropriate to arrange a joint case conference to share valuable information related to their present and future needs.

Withdrawal of professional involvement or discharge should never take place unless adequate arrangements for any continuing care have been agreed and are in place. It is not good practice to withdraw a service or discharge the patient on a Friday or over a weekend. Crises can and do happen and community services are not always easily available at weekends. Patients and relatives feel vulnerable when intensive services are withdrawn. Even though the patient or client may require no immediate intervention, there is a sense of safety or reassurance if it is understood that someone will be available to answer any questions should a problem arise. Ten minutes of therapeutic intervention or discharge preparation pre its withdrawal may save you or another colleague one or more hour's work in crisis follow-up.

It is far more beneficial if the patient or client knows the name of the community, outpatient or other professional who will be providing following-on care. It is more reassuring than, for example, 'the nurse will call sometime next week'.

The procedure for withdrawal of therapeutic intervention or discharge is similar to admission or engagement. When a date is agreed, a multi-copy letter in a simple delete or tick format can be used to record relevant disengagement or discharge information. This should be posted, faxed or e-mailed to the appropriate professional or agency. Do not forget to give the patient or client a copy – this will also help reinforce the information given verbally about others involved in their ongoing care.

Avoiding unnecessary cost and time-wasting

For those who will argue that this is additional bureaucracy gone mad, the above guidance, if acted upon appropriately and carefully followed, is cheaper than the cost of a missed appointment or confusion arising from poor communication. A wasted home visit from a professional colleague or loss of money to the patient from a missed appointment with a benefits agency far outweigh the cost involved in good, effective communication between very busy professionals and agencies.

It is likely that you have already been on the receiving end of such effective action. However, you will probably not have recognised how much time you were saved. Indeed, you may not even be able to recall the event(s). However, it is guaranteed that at some stage during your career, to date, you will on many occasions have experienced frustration from ineffective communication practices. Individual good and bad practices do make a difference, and do affect others.

Once all professionals involved in the care of the patient or client are fully aware of the activities and proposals surrounding the therapeutic interventions on behalf of that individual, there is a reduction in wasted visits and appointments, telephone contact, repetition of tasks and time spent chasing up information.

Being aware of others feelings

Anyone who has made a home visit, only to be greeted by an emotionally distressed relative or friend who informs you that the patient or client died, will recognise the emotional distress this can place on the relative(s) or carer(s). It places an equal effect on you, the professional. Your greeting may have been inappropriate. You will be unprepared to respond to the relative appropriately. If the death is not anticipated, or alternatively your professional interventions have been ongoing for a long time and the patient and carer bond is at a deeper level, you may find the news both distressing and upsetting.

There is very little excuse for such ineffective communication. It is insensitive to the needs of the relative(s) and significant others. It can be, and is, avoidable. If the patient or client dies in hospital, or at home, and you are the community professional involved, it is of vital importance to visit the relative(s) as soon as is practical and inform all other professionals or agencies involved in the care. The visit is essential to enable appropriate support and advice, and to commence closure of the relationship in a therapeutic, caring way.

Effective telecommunication

Effective telecommunication simply means making appropriate use of the telephone to communicate effectively with others. The epidemic of the 'I'll call you back' syndrome grows greater every day. Once the immortal lines have been drawled by the overburdened professional, you can almost guarantee that you will need to re-establish contact later. In other words, chase the person you called. These four words ('I'll call you back') can have a major impact on either the patient or professional colleague on the receiving end of this 'cut off'. It can, and does, leave the caller feeling undervalued.

We all know how frustrating this can be. If, for whatever reason, you are unable to answer a telephone call or cannot deal with the communication immediately, e.g. more research is needed before an appropriate reply can be relayed, do remember to telephone the caller back. If the query is going to take a long time, do make occasional progress calls. This acts as a self-reminder to chase up the query, and lets the originator of the enquiry know it has not been forgotten or undervalued.

It is useful to bear in mind that it may have taken the individual concerned a considerable amount of effort and courage to make the telephone call. Whilst the outcome of the conversation may appear routine to you, it could be of vital importance to the patient, relative(s) or significant others making the call. Equally, it could be you making such a call in the future. Would you like to be treated effectively or to have your query go unanswered and/or misunderstood?

Setting an example to others

Direction on effective communication comes from the top. If the directive shows that clear and effective communication is important, then it is likely that the practice will disseminate effectively to the workforce. However, one cannot place all the responsibility on the boss! Each one of us is capable of demonstrating how communication can be effective if we remain cognisant of the part we all play in ensuring that we are understood and heard. We must also exercise carefully the ability to listen to others and analyse each individual's need. Having done that, no therapeutic intervention can take place unless we act on the information we have, and communicate it to others.

A few minutes spent on effective communication now will save time. Misunderstanding, anger, frustration, complaints and worry can be avoided provided we communicate effectively. Why keep walking into doors? Life is difficult enough! We all have a responsibility to make it easier, not just for ourselves, but for others whose lives we touch in one way or another. Effective communication is the master key. It fits all locks and opens the way to therapeutic caring and interventions.[4]

CHAPTER 19

Conclusion: entering the room

David B Cooper

Alcohol use: a potted history

It is believed that the drinking of alcohol goes as far back as the human race. Possibly one of the earliest mentions of wine-making is dated 3500 BC. Throughout time, alcohol has been central to social, religious and personal use. The making of alcoholic spirits, such as gin and brandy, commenced some 1000 years ago. It has been said that the 'history of drinking is remarkably central to the history of civilisation'.[1] The Romans introduced the vine to England. The Celts introduced the art of distillation to Scotland. European colonists introduced a broad range of alcohol beverages to the Americas, Africa and Australia.

One may assume that with the introduction of alcohol came the excesses and their consequences. Therefore, dealing with alcohol use and related problems is not new. Throughout time, the law has been applied to control the individual whose alcohol use may directly or indirectly affect themselves or others. In 1634, Robert Coles was sentenced for drunkenness. He was committed to prison, disfranchised and forced to wear the letter 'D' round his neck for one year. Failure to wear the 'D' would lead to a fine of 40 shillings for his first offence, and £5 the second offence.[2] In 1636, Peter Busaker fared no better for his public drunkenness; he was given 20 lashes and fined £5.[2]

In the mid 18th and 19th centuries alcohol consumption was high. The production of cheap and strong spirits was much appreciated by the populace. Between 1720 and 1750 the so-called 'gin epidemic' hit Britain. Consumption increased to such a rate that alcohol-related death led the government of the time to pass the 'Gin Act'. The Act placed high taxation on strong spirits in an attempt to discourage its use. The 'Gin Act' is commonly described as becoming law in 1751. However, investigation indicates that the date is incorrect and according to *Jowitt's Dictionary of English Law*,[a] the 'Gin Act' became law in 1735 and is described thus:

'Gin Act, the popular title of the repeated Statute [repealed 1867] 1735, 9 Geo 2, c 23, by which a retailer of spirits in less quantity than two gallons had to pay a licence duty of £50 a year, and a further duty of 20 s, for every gallon sold.'[b]

The 'Gin Act' is the Spirits and Duties Act 1735. However, a copy of the Act obtained from the House of Lords Records Office dates the Act 1736. How much impact the Act had on the gin-consuming populace of the time is unclear. Many saw the upsurge of alcohol consumption during the industrial revolution as a means of escaping the pain and boredom of working life.

Early treatments for alcohol-related problems may cause at least a raised eyebrow today. However, at the time these were claimed to be effective:

- Mullerus (1699)[3] recorded the use of opium or bleeding for treatment of delirium tremens (DTs). The suggested opening for bleeding was the vein in the ham (back of the knee), then the arm and then the forehead (Scarfiy's cupping glass could be applied to the forehead if wished.) Sometimes a vein in the ankle was opened. Drug use included a mixture of waters of male pimpernel, purslain, white water lilies, syrup of water lilies and syrup of poppies. This was used for a 'symptomatical phrensy'. 'Malignant phrensy' required cinnabar of antimony, lunar bezoar, laudanum opiatum and campher. Water of frogs spawn, juice of river-crab, opium dissolved in vinegar, camphyr and saffron were also used.
- Gunn (1859)[4] recorded the use of ether and opium for the treatment of delirium tremens.
- Hartshorne (1871)[5] recorded the use of an infusion of cloves or elixir of valerianate of ammonia for stomach troubles and anxiety following alcohol consumption.
- Chase (1881)[6] recorded that the use of iron, magnesia, peppermint water and spirit of nutmeg would cure the problem of habitual drunkenness.
- Chase (1902)[7] recorded the cure for drunkenness and craving as hemlock bark, cayenne pepper added to tea, bayberry bark, ginger root and cloves.
- Richardson (1909)[8] recorded a 'no fail' cure for drunkenness known as the Keely Gold Cure. This was administered by injection and said to be successful in the case of DTs. The injection contained arsenios acid, tribromide of gold, bromine water and distilled water.

Time has moved on but we remain somewhat committed to the induction of other drugs such as diazepam,[9] chlordiazepoxide[9] and naltrexone,[10] as well as vitamin replacement,[11,12] to control the symptoms produced by withdrawal of alcohol from the body.

Alcohol, its use and alcohol-related problems

Alcohol is the most commonly abused substance in the world.[13] It is the mind-altering substance that we would all like to distance from other mind-altering drugs that are currently illegal in the UK and elsewhere. Once ingested, it begins to induce feelings of well-being and acts as an excellent social lubricant, that is, provided one feels like socialising. As a drug, mixed with human emotion it can also increase feelings of despair to the point of enhancing our individual motivation towards attempting or successfully committing suicide. When alcohol is consumed in large amounts we can behave in ways that are unacceptable to the society in which we live, and yet which often appears accepting of the excuse that we cannot recall our poor behaviour because of its consumption. It is often favourable to 'get blitzed' to the point of physical illness as a means of having 'a good night out'. How one can feel so nauseatingly ill and yet link this to a good time is still a subject for debate.

Alcohol use at a reasonable level, under the correct circumstances, is beneficial, both socially and, there is some indication, physically. However, the use of alcohol causes around 40 000 deaths per annum from overconsumption,[14] it is second to tobacco use as the cause of premature deaths[15] and it is estimated that one in 25 people are dependent on it.[15]

Difficulties arise for the individual when alcohol is used inappropriately. The problem for governments and those working in the research, prevention and treatment fields is that they are working with individuals. As such, to create a general approach to the problems linked to alcohol use, and its associated consequences, in expectation that there will never be any more alcohol-induced problems, is at best unrealistic. Perhaps the best one can do is to keep revising the approach as new information becomes available. Research should lead the way. However, there is no use in funding research if the findings are not transferred into practice, not just by the professional working in the substance use field but the professionals or government who hold a responsibility for the care of individuals within the community, and within society as a whole.

There is, of course, a huge debate about at what point one infringes on civil liberties. Presenting the information and making it available for public consumption is one thing. To dictate can lead to prohibition, and history has demonstrated that this approach does not work. Another factor in the equation is the fact that governments gain great amounts of income from taxation of alcohol products. It is very difficult to do something meaningful if one's income is dependent on the source one wishes to control or lead.

Alcohol and young people

Various steps to control alcohol use among the young adult population are underway in the UK. A Home Office consultation paper[15] proposes that the police be given power to seize alcoholic beverages from the under-age drinker who is found drinking in a public place, and from an adult if it is believed that the alcohol is for an under-age person. Under-age drinkers will be obliged to give their name and address to the police and failure to do so may lead to a fine of £500. The proposal goes as far as to recommend that under-age young adults should be recruited to test the new laws by attempting to purchase alcohol from licensed premises. However, debate and investigation will need to take place as to the legality of this.

The proposals are, of course, one way of approaching the problem of alcohol consumption by the young adult. Nevertheless, acknowledgement should be given to the fact that the young adult does (and has done for many years) consume alcohol before legally entitled to do so. It does not take an expert to walk into a public house and identify young people who are regular attenders. At present, whilst it is an offence for a person under the age of 18 to attempt to buy alcohol and to drink alcohol in a licensed bar, it is not an offence for a child over the age of 5 to drink alcohol in private or public, nor is it an offence for an adult to buy alcohol for consumption by a young adult.

A concerted effort to introduce education on the sensible use of alcohol into schools may be a way forward. The problems encountered by professionals attempting to do so are twofold:

1 Education on the dangers of illegal drugs is encouraged. However, an attempt to introduce education related to sensible alcohol use is not seen as important by many teacher education authorities or consecutive governments
2 If one is invited to put forward an alcohol education package for children and the young adult, the message felt to be acceptable by many schools is one of total abstinence rather than sensible alcohol use.

27% of pupils aged 11–15 were said to have consumed alcohol in the previous week in a survey in 1996, in England, in comparison to 20% in 1988.[16] To ignore the fact that children and young adults are consuming alcohol, which is found to be pleasurable, and expect a resumption of total abstinence is unrealistic. An acknowledgement that some children and young adults do drink alcohol, and will continue to drink alcohol, and a sensible approach to alcohol consumption can be pleasurable but not harmful, is perhaps more realistic. Giving the facts in order to facilitate informed opinion might be the best way of meeting the young adult halfway.

What appears to be a growing concern has yet to find an acceptable, successful approach in terms of prevention of alcohol-related problems. The concept of reducing the legal age limit or removing legislation altogether has yet to be considered. The only thing one can be sure of with the young adult is that the word 'no' generally tends to means 'let's do it!'.[17]

Alcohol and the adult

In Great Britain, in 1998, 39% of men drank more than the four standard drinks in one day and 21% of women drank more than the three standard drinks in one day, currently the 'UK safe limits' for men and women respectively.[16] In 1996, the mean weekly alcohol consumption in Great Britain was 16.6 standard drinks for men and 6.3 standard drinks for women. Alcohol consumption in women drinking over the 14-standard-drink 'UK safe limit', has risen from 10% in 1986 to 14% in 1996.[16] It has been estimated that the annual prevalence rate of alcohol dependence in private households is 75 per 1000 population among men aged 16–64 and 21 per 1000 population among women aged 16–64.[16] During 1997, in Great Britain there were 16 800 casualties in traffic accidents involving illegal alcohol levels. That is 5% of all traffic accidents.[16]

Whilst it is clear that some low-level alcohol consumption can assist in the reduction of some heart problems, it may be that these messages are heard louder than messages related to the adverse effects of excessive alcohol use. It is acknowledged that high levels of alcohol consumption affect women's fertility rates. However, a new report, one of the first, from Denmark suggests that even moderate levels of alcohol consumption (7.5 standard drinks per week) can delay conception in couples who are trying to conceive for the first time.[18] A recent review[19] examining eight studies looked at whether alcohol consumption affects oestrogen levels in post-menopausal women and increases the risk of breast cancer. Excluding women on hormone replacement therapy (HRT) , the review looked at women who drank moderately – 1.5 standard drinks per day. Three of the studies found a relationship between drinking and increased oestrogen levels, but others were inconclusive. Two other studies concluded that, for women on HRT, there was a relation between drinking and increased oestrogen levels. The article concluded that more research was needed in this area. However, it is worth keeping an open mind when advising women in relation to alcohol use. Presentation of knowledge, as it is understood, to the individual is important before informed opinion can take place.

There is an increasing awareness of the link between alcohol use and mental health problems. However, there is also an ever-growing problem in that once the individual with an alcohol and mental health problem is identified there can be difficulty accessing appropriate services for that individual.[20] More work is needed in this neglected area of health, spiritual and social care if the identification and appropriate service provision is to be made for this client group.

When looking at alcohol use and the workforce, one report suggests that an occupation that places few demands on the employee may lead to an increase in alcohol consumption.[21] Alcohol use takes place by employers and employees both within and outwith the workplace on a daily basis at all levels of occupation, within the privatised and nationalised industry as a whole. Workplace policies that facilitate the identification of an individual who may present problems due to their alcohol use are to be encouraged. However, it is essential to ensure that adequate and effective treatment options are available to the identified individual as an integral part of policy implementation. Breathalysing employees as they enter work would be an extreme. However, there is still a need for employers and employees to find a sensible, balanced way forward in making the working environment safer.

It is clear that there is an increasing role for the health, spiritual and social care professional in terms of both prevention and identification of alcohol-related problems. Much has been written about the need for education and training of these professionals. One initiative in formative process at the time of writing is the development of a national charity under the name of the *Nursing Council on Alcohol and Drugs (NCAD)*. Supported by leading nurses, the aim is to develop a registered charity with openly elected trustees. This will be an apolitical organisation. That is, it is not about applying political pressure. However, it will be willing to offer its best consultative guidance and advice if requested. The sole aim is to raise awareness of alcohol and drug-related problems at a UK level. Working along the lines established by the Medical Council on Alcoholism (MCA), it is envisaged that there will be a committee of leaders in the field who will direct their energies towards raising awareness, and providing advice and information, to the nursing profession – organisations or individuals – the concept being that raised awareness leads to improved, early identification of alcohol and drug-related problems, and the consequential provision of adequate and appropriate intervention at the entrance point to nursing care, which will assist in the reduction of costly interventions at a later time. The aim is to establish national and regional contacts that are ready and willing to provide support, advice and information. Those individuals will monitor and provide active intervention on educational needs at a national, regional and local level.

This is, of course, a brief outline of the vision. Such initiatives are to be encouraged. However, they do need the support of the nursing profession as a whole. Direction needs to come from the top, at the same time encouraging a 'bottom-up' approach in the way that information and knowledge can be shared.

Action for the policy makers

About every 10 years in the UK, the government pays a visit to the issues related to alcohol use problems encountered by the individual. Because action in this area is not a popular vote catcher, much is promised but little is done! Such a review is taking place as this chapter is written. Alcohol Concern[22] continues to argue for a national strategy to ensure policy is given a high priority. The call is for a move away from the current, inappropriate tagging of alcohol issues on to drug policy.

Successive government strategies have highlighted alcohol as a causative factor in priority diseases, e.g. coronary heart disease, stroke, cancer, mental illness and accident.[23,24] The 1999 public health strategy[24] made a commitment to encouraging sensible drinking habits on the provision of services of 'proven effectiveness' to enable people to overcome alcohol use.

Some move is anticipated in terms of legislation related to drink-driving. An opinion poll carried out by a UK magazine[25] suggested that 82% of people are in favour of a lower drink-drive limit (52% in favour of zero limit, 27% in favour of 50 mg percentage limit). 26% felt that the zero limit would be unfair to those living in remote areas; however, 60% thought that public outrage would be reduced by a zero limit.[25]

The British Medical Association (BMA) is currently leading the call for a reduction in the legal blood alcohol limit for driving. The call is for a reduction from 80 mg per 100 ml of blood to 50 mg per 100 ml blood. In its report,[26] which is supported by the cross-party Parliamentary Advisory Council for Transport Safety (PACT) and Alcohol Concern, it is noted that seven of the 15 members of the European Union (EU) countries already have this level and that the move to decrease the limit to 50 mg per 100 ml of blood would assist in harmonisation of the legal drink-drive limits in the EU. It is suggested that such a reduction could lead to 500 fewer deaths per annum on UK roads.[26] Lowering the legal drink-drive limit to 50 mg per 100 ml is also central to a government consultative paper.[27] However, an article published in *Alcoholism*[28] goes one step further – though it agrees with a reduction in the legal limit, it also argues for a concerted prevention programme. It suggests that as a practical approach to early intervention it should be recognised that a significant proportion of high-risk drink-drivers are young adults, and proposes that individuals who have recently passed their test should be required to receive mandatory screening and education about drink-driving.[28]

In Germany, since the introduction of the 0.5 mg percentage drink-drive limit on 1 May 1998, the number of alcohol-related accidents in Cologne is claimed to have halved. According to the German Office of National Statistics (Das Statistische Bundesamt), the overall number of accidents involving drivers who have consumed alcohol has also fallen.[29] The Spanish government also reduced its drink-drive levels in October 1999 to 0.5 mg percentage, and 0.3 mg percentage for professional drivers.[30] Given this, and the encouraging noises that appear to be stemming from within the UK government, it seems likely that the UK drink-drive limits will be lowered.

On 11 May 1999, the Home Office indicated that a provisional timetable for consultation on licensing legislation will probably be issued in Spring 2000.[31] Current licensing is considered by some to be cumbersome and out of date. The Home Office is said to be committed to carrying out a major review. Even if this timetable is adhered to and parliamentary time found, it is unlikely that legislation will be in place much before 2002.

On 26 May 1999, the government announced its timetable for the new strategy to tackle alcohol misuse. Due for publication in the summer of 1999, publication is still awaited at the time of writing this chapter.[32]

Such legislation is good provided it is funded and can be realistically translated into practice. This naturally requires government will. Those who remember the 'Kessel Reports', published in 1978 and 1979,[33–35] will know that many good recommendations can be left to collect dust if funding and resources are not encouraged and made available. Targets to reduce a figure are fine provided that the means by which this can be achieved are active, current, in place and under constant review and revision. At the same time, service provision needs to be available, and effective, for those individuals who choose to continue to consume alcohol that may lead them or others into problems.

Reflection

Referring back to the house purchaser analogy used in Chapter 1, 'Introduction: opening the door', it is hoped that you have found the basic contents of this book helpful and informative. One would wish that the reader feels sufficiently stimulated to proceed, having extended and developed their knowledge and understanding of alcohol use and alcohol-related problems, and that this leads to incorporation of effective alcohol interventions and practice into everyday professional activity.

Now that the basics have been explored, each chapter can be built upon, using the 'To learn more' sections of the book as a guide to further study and knowledge. As one enters each new area of knowledge (each new room), so understanding improves. With that comes the ability to use a holistic and eclectic approach to the problems identified by the individual presenting for intervention, advice or treatment.

As we enter each room or if we choose to purchase the property in the analogy, we discover more about its past and its future. One thing that is certain is that we will never know all there is to know about the house, and it will always offer up surprises. So it is with working with the individual who, for one reason or another, is experiencing problems resultant from his or another person's use of alcohol. What we do at that point depends on our knowledge and our ability to use other people's knowledge, whatever that may be. We have a responsibility to offer the best that we know of, to the best of our ability, at that time.

Our knowledge and understanding of alcohol use is constantly changing. The challenge is to remain open to the information that will help each one of us provide appropriate therapeutic intervention:

- at the appropriate level
- at the appropriate time
- at the appropriate cost
- with the appropriate understanding of the individual presenting with the problem.

It is a waste of all we know to work in the cocoon of belief that all individuals are the same.

This book does not contain all the answers. It will not make the reader an 'expert'. If it encourages the reader to learn more, then it has achieved its aim. If it helps the reader to at least appreciate and understand some of the problems related to alcohol and its use encountered by some individuals, then it has 'opened the door'. One hopes that the reader will progress to enter each room – and purchase the property!

To develop your knowledge in this area, see 'To learn more', pp. 273–5.

Notes

a The author is indebted to Jackie, Senior Office Clerk, House of Commons Information Office, for her work in tracking down the 'Gin Act' and checking its accuracy. Her co-operation and guidance is much appreciated. Thank you also to John Breslin, House of Lords Records Office.

   'AD 1736. Anno 9° GeorgII. c 19–23. pp 431–9. CAP XXIII. An Act for laying a Duty upon the Retailers of Spirituous Liquors, and for licencing the Retailer thereof.'

b Jowitt, Earl Rt Hon and Walsh C (1977) *Jowitt's Dictionary of English Law* (2nd edn by J Burke [Barrister, sometime Editor of *Current Law*]. 2nd impression [1990], p. 860.) Sweet & Maxwell Ltd, London.

Reader questionnaire

The editor and authors are keen to hear from readers of this book – your comments and opinions are important to us. Book reviews are very helpful but the views of the reader give a more helpful indication of the value of a book. The questionnaire below can be photocopied and returned to the book editor. It is completely confidential.

Your help is appreciated. Thank you.

1   When did you purchase this book? ....

2   Where did you purchase this book? ....

3   Was the book too long, too short, just right? ....

4   What did you most enjoy about the book? ....

5   What did you least enjoy about the book? ....

6   What did you learn? ....

    ....

7   What did you not learn? ....

    ....

8   What would you like to see included in any revision of this book? ....

    ....

9   What would you like excluded from any revision of this book? ....

    ....

10 Which chapter did you like best? ....

10a Why? ....

    ....

    ....

11 Which chapter did you like least? ....

11a Why? ....

    ....

    ....

12 Did the book achieve its stated aims? ....

12a If yes, how? ....

....

12b If no, why? ....

....

13 How, in your opinion, could the book be improved? ....

....

14 What is your profession and occupation? ....

....

15 What courses are you currently studying, or expecting to study? ....

....

16 Please feel free to add any additional comments you feel may be helpful to the
    editor and authors ....

....

....

....

....

....

....

....

....

Please return the questionnaire to:

Mr David B Cooper
Parkholme
Ashreigney
Chulmleigh
Devon
EX18 7LY
UK

Thank you for your help. Completion of this questionnaire will entitle you to a reduction
of £10 off the annual subscription to the *Journal of Substance Use*.

Answers to self-assessment questions

Chapter 3

1 10 millilitres.
2 Factors include:
- the personality characteristics of the drinker
- the mood of the drinker before they start consuming
- the expectancies they bring into the drinking occasion
- their reasons for wishing to drink
- the site of consumption
- the company or lack of it
- the behaviour of those surrounding the drinker
- time of day.
3 According to McKechnie,[2] there are at least four definitions of *drunk*:
- the emotional state produced by any level of alcoholisation
- the emotional state produced by extreme degrees of alcoholisation
- the behaviour produced by extreme degrees of alcoholisation
- a retrospective definition based on subsequent events. 'I must have been drunk because ..., I've got a hangover, I don't remember what happened ..., I fell over on the dance floor ...'.
4 Functional drinking is where the purpose of drinking is internal and not social; it is to alter personal mental state rather than to facilitate social interaction.
5 According to Mulford,[6] drinkers are more likely to be labelled problem drinkers or 'alcoholics' if the drinking is:
- causing trouble
- functional (personal effects drinking)
- central (preoccupied drinking)
- uncontrolled.

Chapter 4

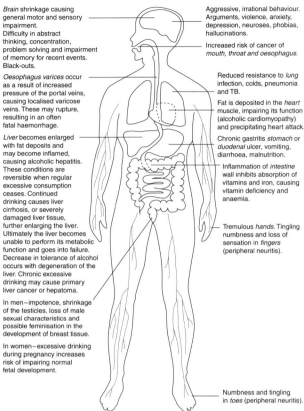

Brain shrinkage causing general motor and sensory impairment. Difficulty in abstract thinking, concentration, problem solving and impairment of memory for recent events. Black-outs.

Oesophagus varices occur as a result of increased pressure of the portal veins, causing localised varicose veins. These may rupture, resulting in an often fatal haemorrhage.

Liver becomes enlarged with fat deposits and may become inflamed, causing alcoholic hepatitis. These conditions are reversible when regular excessive consumption ceases. Continued drinking causes liver cirrhosis, or severely damaged liver tissue, further enlarging the liver. Ultimately the liver becomes unable to perform its metabolic function and goes into failure. Decrease in tolerance of alcohol occurs with degeneration of the liver. Chronic excessive drinking may cause primary liver cancer or hepatoma.

In men – impotence, shrinkage of the testicles, loss of male sexual characteristics and possible feminisation in the development of breast tissue.

In women – excessive drinking during pregnancy increases risk of impairing normal fetal development.

Aggressive, irrational behaviour. Arguments, violence, anxiety, depression, neuroses, phobias, hallucinations.

Increased risk of cancer of *mouth, throat and oesophagus.*

Reduced resistance to *lung* infection, colds, pneumonia and TB.

Fat is deposited in the *heart* muscle, impairing its function (alcoholic cardiomyopathy) and precipitating heart attack.

Chronic gastritis *stomach* or *duodenal* ulcer, vomiting, diarrhoea, malnutrition.

Inflammation of *intestine* wall inhibits absorption of vitamins and iron, causing vitamin deficiency and anaemia.

Tremulous *hands*. Tingling numbness and loss of sensation in *fingers* (peripheral neuritis).

Numbness and tingling in *toes* (peripheral neuritis).

1 Ethyl alcohol, ethanol (commonly used in North America). C_2H_5OH is the chemical formula, where C = carbon, H = hydrogen and O = oxygen.

2 It is a sedative and analgesic.

3 Cultural, environmental and genetic.

4 30 mg per 100 ml.

5 Dehydrogenases, which oxidise alcohol into other chemicals.

6 Eight hours – the liver disposes of approximately 1 standard drink per hour.

7 Keep within recommended weekly limits, but note that as little as one to two standard drinks two or three times a week is protective.

8 Excess alcohol is converted via lactic acid to uric acid; deposition of the latter around joints causes gout in susceptible individuals.

9 Tremor, agitation, sweating, insomnia, confusion.

10 Peripheral neuropathy, Wernicke's encephalopathy, Korsakoff's syndrome, beri-beri heart failure.

11 Hypoglycaemia (low blood sugar) because of insufficient stores of glycogen in the liver.

Chapter 5

1   21.
2   b.
3   c.
4   Yes.
5   Yes.
6   Yes.
7   To periodic heavy drinking and intoxication.
8   A higher risk.
9   Strong.
10 Yes.

Chapter 6

1 Yes. Men are drinking less and women more. See 'History'.
2 Yes. From concentrating upon public drunkenness by men to consumption levels and drinking patterns by all drinkers. See 'History'.
3 Yes. Different attitudes of responsibility, control and image. See 'History' and 'Men and women: differences in drinking'.
4 No. In all recorded drinking cultures, men drink more than women. See 'History'.
5 Divorce, separation, never married, homosexuality. See 'Men and women: similarities'.
6 No. See 'Women: gender-specific issues'.
7 Men. See 'Women: gender-specific issues' and 'Men: gender-specific issues'.
8 No. See 'Gender differences in response to treatment'.
9 Women. See 'Gender differences in response to treatment'.
10 Yes. See 'Employment'.

Chapter 7

1   Some of the main difficulties that alcohol problems can cause for family members include:
*   family members often suffer many negative experiences, including violence, poverty and social isolation
*   family members will often develop problems because of these experiences
*   some will be individual problems (such as anxiety and depression)
*   others will be family problems (such as breakdowns in such family structures and systems as rituals, roles, routines, communication structures, social life and finances)
*   children may have particular difficulties, demonstrating whilst still young a higher propensity for antisocial behaviour, emotional problems and problems in the school environment, and during adolescence often showing friendship difficulties, a division between home life and peer relationships, being prescribed psychoactive drugs, earlier use of alcohol or drugs, leaving home early, earlier marriages and involvement with a 'semi-deviant' subculture.

2   There are often problems in:
*   family rituals
*   family roles
*   family routines
*   family communication
*   family social life
*   family finances.

3   The key issues that make a bad situation worse are:
*   **violence**: even if it is not directed at the child
*   **marital conflict**: the major concern of the child
*   **separation, divorce and parent loss**
*   **inconsistency and ambivalence in parenting**
*   all of these elements lead to **unpredictability**, which leads to many other difficulties:
    – a deteriorating parent–child relationship
    – diminishing feelings of self-esteem
    – social isolation
    – feelings of exclusion.

4   The key protective issues which often lead to resilience are:
    For children
*   how the parent without the drinking problem reacts
*   the extent to which the parents still maintain a cohesive parental relationship
*   the extent to which the family still maintains a cohesive family relationship

- the extent to which the family can maintain a family life which is separate from the disruptive behaviour of the problem drinker
- other important influences – a non-parental adult such as a grandparent, an influential teacher or a neighbour
- the extent to which the child can disengage from the disruptive elements of family life, and engage with stabilising activities or other people outside the family
- the development of 'planning' or 'deliberateness' – the active and deliberate attempt to make one's life more ordered and structured, and less disrupted by the problems in the family.
  For adults
- the development or continuation of 'planning' or 'deliberateness' – the active and deliberate attempt to make one's life more ordered and structured, and less disrupted by the problems in the family
- the selection of a stable partner
- the formation of a new family
- the deliberate attempt to select positive family rituals.

5 Children (and most adults) need **attachment** and **security** as opposed to unpredictability, insecurity, exclusion and isolation. Stability allows children to grow and explore their environments, secure in the knowledge that parent figures are there to help and offer support when challenges or problems are met. Without that stability, children either become fearful of this necessary exploration, or develop problems when they do meet challenges and have no one to help them work through them.

6 The main ways family members can be helped include:
- designated services for children
- specialised child and family workers within Alcohol Services
- specialised alcohol workers within Child & Family Services
- offering a confidential service for children such that they can develop sufficient confidence and security to clarify how to deal with their problems in their own time.

7 The key skills needed to help family members are:
- to be warm, empathic and genuine
- to develop a therapeutic relationship
- to help family members explore their difficulties
- to enable family members to set achievable goals
- to empower family members to take action to reach these achievable goals
- to maintain therapeutic contact with family members and help them stabilise and maintain their changed behaviours, their changed thoughts, and their changed emotions, which will have come about through the process of helping.

Chapter 8

List of indicators that appear in case study 2

Because there are symptoms of ageing that can mimic alcohol consumption problems, and vice versa, there is a strong need for a thorough assessment in order to avoid both a misdiagnosis and a missed opportunity to intervene. For instance, the cut on the forehead suggests a contusion, memory impairment suggests dementia and swollen abdomen may suggest the need for further investigation other than alcohol-induced oedema. Confusion, coordination and slurred speech could have one of several causes that need to be investigated appropriately.

With this broader perspective in mind, the following is a list of indicators of a potential addiction problem:

- confusion
- poor hygiene
- weight loss (report from wife and observations that sandwich is uneaten)
- slurred speech
- alcohol odour
- laceration on forehead
- oedema
- 'punk' could be interpreted as flu-like symptoms
- 'so, what's the difference anyway?' could be interpreted as an indication of depression
- coordination problems with the television remote; wife compensating by completing action
- nesting in his chair, with need to be mobile minimised
- 'early retirement' begs the question: 'was it drinking-related?'

Author's response to self-assessment question

Developing our own professional knowledge base on this issue is the fundamental groundwork that is needed and that will serve us well when pursuing subsequent steps. Examples of areas in which to pursue additional knowledge are listed below. This list is by no means exhaustive. The material in most of these areas is immense. Since this chapter is set in the context of a book on alcohol use, this response focuses on ageing specific areas for development. Your existing knowledge base, your professional setting and your developmental goals will all determine your action plan.

Creative and efficient strategies to increase our knowledge base include discussion sessions with colleagues on a chosen reading or topic. This strategy increases the probability that:

- we will benefit from others' perspectives
- solutions to better serve this population will be given group support.

Suggested areas to explore include:

- normal ageing from biological, psychological and sociological perspectives
- loss, grief and adaptation
- psychodynamics of ageing
- clinical syndromes and their assessment (i.e. depression, dementia, delirium, paranoid disorders, substance use problems)
- management of difficult behaviours (i.e. sleep disturbances, wandering, sexual disinhibition, incontinence, paranoid symptoms, hostility and aggression, driving, communication and the mentally impaired client)
- medication problems (i.e. psychotropic medication, antidepressants, lithium carbonate, major tranquillisers, anxiolytics and hypnotics)
- elder abuse (i.e. definitions, causes, assessment, interventions)
- legal issues (i.e. refusal of services, financial incompetence and guardianship)
- family ties and ageing: family dynamics, family therapy
- nutrition, substance use and the older person.

Developing this knowledge base is an ongoing task and the hallmark of a professional. The implementation of this developing knowledge base into change includes examining our own employment environment for its suitability to address this issue. For instance:

- physical barriers to accessing treatment

- policy barriers such as age restrictions
- the percentage of resource material and time that is allocated to this population
- marketing resources that target this population.

By exploring change at these levels, we may have an impact on changes within systems.

Chapter 9

1 Yes. For example, people with a history of major depression or anxiety have double the risk in comparison with the general population. Approximately 50% of young people with schizophrenia or bipolar affective disorder are likely to have a significant problem with alcohol or other drugs. The reasons vary for individuals: the same reasons other people in the community use alcohol; as an attempt to alleviate the symptoms of mental illness; to reduce side-effects of medication.

2 Yes. Alcohol is recognised as a problematic substance for a person's mental health. Most significant risks are depression and suicide; however, when alcohol is used problematically a person is more vulnerable to a wide range of mental health problems.

3 There are three clear groups of problems: separate systems, a lack of education and training, and a lack of tailored and flexible treatment programmes.

4 (i) An integrated approach – combining the principles of mental health treatment and drug and alcohol treatment. (ii) There is a need to improve education and training about the other system of care (i.e. improved education and training for mental health professionals about alcohol use and treatment, and training for drug and alcohol treatment providers about mental illness and treatment). (iii) A more flexible and tailored treatment programme is required (e.g. particularly for people who need a comprehensive range of services, a longer period of treatment or find it extremely difficult to commit to abstinence).

5 Biological, psychological, educational and social interventions.

6 Engagement, persuasion, active treatment and relapse prevention.

7 The engagement stage is generally considered the most challenging stage. There are many reasons why a person may not be easily engaged in the treatment programme:

- There may be more important needs which have to be addressed first (e.g. assistance with housing, food and clothing; healthcare; provision of legal advice or referral; social and vocational opportunities). These basic human needs will often be a person's priority.

- Trusting and liking a therapist (and therapy) is a process which takes time – be prepared for this.

- Therapy is orientated towards change – does the person want to change and what exactly does the person want to change? These questions need to be asked and then matched to the therapist's concept of therapy.

8 During the engagement stage it is important not to make strong demands on the person to stop or reduce alcohol use. The engagement

stage needs to be alluring and non-threatening. It is acceptable for the therapist to indicate their disapproval of excessive alcohol intake.

9   People with mental illnesses can and do have relapses. People with alcohol problems can and do have relapses. The key to therapy for these problems is to anticipate and prepare for relapse. Identify early warning signs of relapse and identify plans to reduce the risk of relapse. Identify a plan if relapse occurs and recognise this is a process of treatment as opposed to failure. Maintain a positive outlook and a long-term focus (as well as a short-term focus) during relapses.

Chapter 12

1   Problem drinking affects:
*   the person him/herself
*   the person's family
*   the person's colleagues and employer
*   members of society through alcohol-related accidents, and the costs of legal, social and healthcare resources.

2   Success in reducing the amount of alcohol which everyone drinks can help to reduce alcohol-related problems by a relatively greater proportion. This is because the majority of alcohol-related disability is caused by moderate drinkers, rather than the relatively small number of individuals who are habitual heavy drinkers. Achievement of a reduction in consumption by everyone would result in a high proportion of people who are currently at a moderate risk (i.e. above the sensible limits) moving to a low risk (i.e. to within the sensible limits). As their levels of consumption fall, so also will the frequency with which they experience alcohol-related problems.

3   The Health Education Authority's recommended limits for sensible drinking are 21 standard drinks per week for men, and 14 standard drinks per week for women.

4   (i)   False. One pint of 4.5% alcohol by volume (ABV) beer contains 2.6 standard drinks of alcohol.
     (ii) False. One can of extra-strong lager contains four standard drinks, i.e. the equivalent of *two* double measures of whisky.
     (iii) True. One bottle of 8% ABV table wine contains six standard drinks of alcohol.
     (iv) True. One standard drink of alcohol is contained in 25 ml of spirits.

5   Everyone should have at least two alcohol-free days each week.

6   A retrospective diary is preferable because it enables one to gain much more information than is possible from quantity and frequency measures. Quantity and frequency measures are calculated by asking how much and how often a person drinks, and then multiplying the two numbers. Patterns of alcohol consumption, such as drinking which tends to be concentrated on certain days of the week (e.g. at weekends), cannot therefore be noted. Since many people do not drink the same amount on each occasion, it is very likely that errors could be made using this method.

Using a diary also helps to identify what kinds of alcohol the person drinks. This information can be used to form the basis of advice regarding how to cut down, if this is deemed appropriate. For example, someone who says that they drink 6% ABV beer can be encouraged to achieve a substantial reduction by opting to drink 3.5% ABV beer instead. It is also possible to assess where and with whom the person drinks, which can be useful when planning ways of cutting down.

Chapter 13

1   d.
2   c.
3   d.
4   a.
5   b.

Chapter 14

1 Anyone can do an assessment of another person's drinking! In the caring professions a whole range of primary, secondary and tertiary care workers have a responsibility to make such assessments. However, they do not all need to assess the same things in the same way. Assessments by primary care professionals often focus around clarifying whether referral to a specialist is indicated. Specialists usually assess to determine what sort of treatment or other help to offer.

2 Definitions vary, but screening is usually used to describe the process of identifying any individuals in a given group whose drinking is already or potentially problematic. Assessment usually describes what happens next, when those individuals are interviewed and or examined to clarify the exact nature of the problems with a view to agreeing a way forward.

3 People are most likely to be honest when the consequences of such honesty are expected to be beneficial or neutral. Dishonesty is frequently a form of self-preservation in a situation perceived to be threatening. Both the context of the assessment and the demeanour and skills of the interviewer will thus be crucial. In addition, straight answers are more likely to be given to straight questions. The answer to *'would you call yourself a social drinker?'* may be less helpful than the answer to *'how much did you drink each day last week?'* if the purpose of the question was to ascertain whether the person drinks heavily.

4 It can be extremely helpful to spend 20 minutes or more talking in a focused way about an aspect of one's lifestyle, especially to someone who is interested and sufficiently well informed to prompt with relevant questions. Behaviours such as drinking are often so woven into the fabric of our social lives and coping mechanisms that it can feel as if they are automatic, that no decision-making is involved. It is only when problems are identified that we are invited to reflect on them and this gives us the chance to re-evaluate the many small decisions that make up a habit or even a dependence. It is also helpful and illuminating to hear ourselves describe our lives to someone else. 'Seeing yourself as others see you' can prompt change in itself.

5 Only you have the answer to this question but it is a crucial one and the answer may not always be the same. It will be inseparable from your understanding of your professional responsibilities to the client and the current resources and priorities of your agency.

Chapter 15

1 See Box 15.1, p. 174.
2 People with a regular alcohol intake of 80–100 grams (8–10 standard drinks per day) or more should be considered to be at risk of withdrawing in the event of abstinence. 10 grams of alcohol is approximately equal to one standard drink. The severity of withdrawals is likely to be increased if a person has:
- previous severe withdrawals
- comorbidity, such as epilepsy, hypertension, cardiomyopathy, hepatitis, pancreatitis, pneumonia or a psychiatric condition.[5]
3 A comprehensive client assessment should include:
- quantity, frequency and duration of alcohol use
- time of the last drink
- use of other drugs, prescribed and non-prescribed
- previous withdrawal episodes
- medical conditions (epilepsy, hypertension, pancreatitis, blood-borne viruses, peptic ulcer, trauma, peripheral neuropathy, liver disease) and psychiatric conditions (schizophrenia, affective disorders, anxiety, psychosis, suicidal ideation, previous psychological treatment, etc.)
- social stressors (legal, relationships, job, financial problems)
- breathalyser reading
- level of dependence on alcohol.
4 See Box 15.2, p. 177.
5 The risk factors that must be considered when assessing people for withdrawal in the home are related to the individual and the setting.

Individual
In addition to the factors itemised under 'Assessment', information should be obtained on the following:
- failure to complete previous home or out-patient-based withdrawal
- geographical and social isolation.

Setting
When assessing the suitability of the home as a setting for withdrawal, the Home Environment Assessment (HEA) is a useful tool.[7] On a range of 0–3 this scale allows a quantifiable assessment of the:
- availability of a support person
- attitude of the support person
- commitment of the supporter
- presence of young children and or pets
- general atmosphere and level of noise in the home
- presence of other drinkers.

All these factors have a strong influence on how withdrawal will be experienced in the home. The maximum score on the scale is 24, and high scores indicate that the home setting is likely to be unsuitable for withdrawal. Comprehensive guidelines for home withdrawal have been produced.[7,17]

Chapter 16

1 Treatment should be viewed as a system or process that may take many forms and include many interventions. Some of these interventions may be provided by specialist alcohol or other drug services, others may be provided by general community services. Yet other interventions may be provided by self-help groups such as AA.

2 The main stages of treatment are detoxification, rehabilitation/follow-up and maintenance.

3 The counselling currently recommended combines the basic skills described by Egan[8] in combination with the components of motivational interviewing. For a recent description of motivational interviewing, see Noonan and Moyers.[12]

4 Alcohol problems do not occur in a vacuum; neither does treatment. A comprehensive assessment is multidimensional. It needs to take into account the following:

The client
- presenting problem
- alcohol and other drug use history
- previous treatment
- health, psychological/psychiatric status
- legal problems
- drinking goals.
  The client's social environment
- family structure
- social support
- use of leisure.

Remember assessment is not a one-off event. It is ongoing throughout treatment, and should inform treatment.

5 Access to services may be limited by:
- time – the service may only be available during the day. If the client is working full time and is not able to arrange time out to attend, such a service will not be an option. Alternatively, the service concerned may have a waiting list and it may not be possible to access it when needed
- distance – services are not available in the vicinity
- cost – services are available but the client cannot afford the price
- client preference – services are available but the client does not care for some aspects of the way they are provided. The flip side of this is if a client has been disruptive in a previous treatment episode, they may find that they are denied access. This is not common but has been known to occur.

Chapter 17

1   False. Interdisciplinary interactions are those in which different disciplines support solutions and create common ground by transcending their discipline-specific boundaries.

2   A group becomes a team when each member of each discipline feels they can safely share, trust that their professional boundaries will not be eroded and are able to recognise and respect the skill of others.

3   True. To ensure effective, efficient and appropriate responses to patient needs, team members must have clarity about their relative role and responsibilities.

4   A true interdisciplinary approach relies on the competence and mastery of discipline-specific knowledge, expertise and accountability, as well as a willingness to share in the development of common ground.

5   The advantages of interdisciplinary education and service delivery are:
*   sharing of viewpoints from a variety of backgrounds
*   increased resources and a shared workload
*   increased skills and abilities for addressing complex projects, problems and questions
*   the provision of opportunities for individuals to develop and broaden personal networks
*   sharing in the reward of a successful mutual endeavour.

References/To learn more

Preface

1 Grant M (ed) (1998) *Alcohol in Emerging Markets*. Brunner/Mazel, Philadelphia.
2 Cameron D (1995) *Liberating Solutions to Alcohol Problems: treating problem drinkers without saying no*. Jason Aronson, Northvale, New Jersey.
3 Plant MA, Single E and Stockwell T (eds) (1997) *Alcohol: minimising the harm*. Free Association Books, London.
4 Royal College of Psychiatrists (1986) *Alcohol: our favourite drug*. Tavistock, London.
5 Cooper DB (1994) *Alcohol Home Detoxification and Assessment*. Radcliffe Medical Press, Oxford.

Chapter 2

1 Stockwell T and Single E (1997) Standard unit labelling of alcohol containers. In *Alcohol: minimising the harm* (eds M Plant, E Single and T Stockwell). Free Association Books Ltd, London.
2 Data provided by Centre for Information on Beverage Alcohol. See also AIM, 1996, **5**(2): 11; ICAP *Reports 1* (Supplement), 1996.
3 Data provided by CBA.
4 *South China Morning Post*. 19 September 1996.
5 Jernigan DH (1997) *Thirsting for Markets: the global impact of corporate alcohol*. The Marin Institute, San Rafael, CA.
6 United States Department of Agriculture/United States Department of Health and Human Services (USDA/USD-HHS) (1995) *Nutrition and Your Health: dietary guidelines for Americans* (4th edn). USGPO, Washington, DC.
7 Turner C (1990) How much alcohol is in a 'standard drink'? An analysis of 125 studies. *British Journal of Addiction*. **85**: 1171–5.
8 Wechsler H, Davenport A, Dowdall G *et al*. (1994) Health and behavioral consequences of binge drinking in college: a national survey of students at 140 campuses. *Journal of the American Medical Association*. **272**: 1672–7; International Center for Alcohol Policies (1997) *ICAP Reports 2: The limits of binge drinking*. ICAP, Washington, DC.
9 Williams GD, Deitz DK and Campbell KE (1997) *Frequency of consuming 5+ vs. 9+ drinks a day as predictors of alcohol-related morbidity*. Paper presented at International Workshop on Consumption Measures and Models for Use in Policy Development and Evaluation, 12–14 May, Bethesda, Maryland.

10 Stockwell T and Stirling L (1989) Estimating alcohol contents of drinks: common errors in applying the unit system. *British Medical Journal*. **298**: 271–2.

11 Lemmens RH (1994) The alcohol content of self-report and 'standard' drinks. *Addiction*. **89**: 593–601.

Chapter 3

1 MacAndrew C and Edgerton R (1969) *Drunken Comportment: a social explanation*. Aldine, Chicago.

2 McKechnie RJ (1980) Who's drunk, or whose drunk? In *Aspects of Alcohol and Drug Dependence* (eds JS Madden, R Walker and WH Kenyon). Pitman Medical, Tunbridge Wells.

3 McKechnie RJ (1984) Normal problems with alcohol use. *New Directions in the Study of Alcohol Group Booklet No. 8*, pp. 75–86. (Informal publication of the group.)

4 Kilty KM (1983) Styles of drinking and types of drinker. *Journal of Studies on Alcohol*. **44**: 797–916.

5 Cameron D (1995) *Liberating Solutions to Alcohol Problems: treating problem drinkers without saying no*. Jason Aronson, Northvale, NJ.

6 Mulford HA (1977) Stages in the alcoholic process: towards a cumulative non-sequential index. *Journal of Studies on Alcohol*. **38**: 563–83.

Chapter 3 : To learn more

These three texts are all substantial and erudite. None of them is an 'easy read' but they all contribute significantly to our understanding of drinkers and drinking.

Cox WM (ed) (1990) *Why People Drink: parameters of alcohol as a reinforcer*. Gardner Press, New York.

Pittman DJ and White HR (eds) (1991) *Society, Culture and Drinking Patterns Re-examined*. Rutgers Center of Alcohol Studies, New Brunswick, NJ.
(This is an update of a 1962 classic text, *Society, Culture and Drinking Patterns*, by DJ Pittman and CR Snyder.)

Plant ML (1997) *Women and Alcohol: contemporary and historical perspectives*. Free Association Books, London.

This anthology gives many quotations and extracts from mostly English-speaking literature. It is non-scientific and illuminating.

Rae S (ed) (1991) *The Faber Book Of Drink, Drinkers and Drinking*. Faber & Faber, London.

Chapter 4

1 Keller M (1979) A historical overview of alcohol and alcoholism. *Cancer Research.* **39**: 2822–9.

2 Sournia J-C (1990) *A History of Alcoholism.* Basil Blackwell, Oxford.

3 Clifford CA, Hopper JL, Fulker DW *et al.* (1984) A genetic and environmental analysis of a twin study of alcohol use, anxiety and depression. *Genetic Epidemiology.* **1**: 63–79.

4 Jones BM and Jones MK (1976) Women and alcohol: intoxication, metabolism and the menstrual cycle. In *Alcoholism Problems in Women and Children* (eds M Greenblatt and M Schuckit), pp. 103–36. Grune & Stratton, New York.

5 Paton A (1989) Alcohol misuse and the hospital doctor. *British Journal of Hospital Medicine.* **42**: 394–9.

6 Ashworth M and Gerada C (1997) Addiction and dependence – II: Alcohol. *British Medical Journal.* **315**: 358–60.

7 Rimm EB, Klatsky A, Grobbee D *et al.* (1996) Review of moderate alcohol consumption and reduced risk of coronary heart disease: is the effect due to beer, wine, or spirits? *British Medical Journal.* **312**: 731–6.

8 Marmot MG, Elliott P, Shipley MJ *et al.* (1994) Alcohol and blood pressure: the INTERSALT study. *British Medical Journal.* **308**: 1263–7.

9 World Hypertension League (1991) Alcohol and hypertension – implications for management. *Journal of Human Hypertension.* **5**: 227–32.

10 Anderson P, Cremona A, Paton A *et al.* (1993) The risk of alcohol. *Addiction.* **88**: 1493–508.

11 Ammann RW, Heitz PU and Klöppel G (1996) Course of alcoholic chronic pancreatitis: a clinicomorphological long-term study. *Gastroenterology.* **111**: 224–31.

12 Sherlock S (1995) Alcoholic liver disease. *Lancet.* **345**: 227–9.

13 Sharpe PC, McBride R and Archbold GPR (1996) Biochemical markers of alcohol abuse. *Quarterly Journal of Medicine.* **89**: 137–44.

14 Charness ME, Simon RP and Greenberg DA (1989) Ethanol and the nervous system. *New England Journal of Medicine.* **321**: 442–54.

15 Brennan FN and Lyttle JA (1987) Alcohol and seizures: a review. *Journal of the Royal Society of Medicine.* **80**: 571–3.

16 Gill JS, Zezulka AV, Shipley MJ *et al.* (1986) Stroke and alcohol consumption. *New England Journal of Medicine.* **315**: 1041–6.

17 Ron MA, Acker W, Shaw GK and Lishman WA (1982) Computerized tomography of the brain in chronic alcoholism. A survey and follow-up study. *Brain.* **105**: 497–514.

18 Sillaupää ML (1992) Treatment of alcohol withdrawal symptoms. *British Journal of Hospital Medicine.* **45**: 343–50.

19 Harper CG, Giles M and Finlay-Jones R (1986) Clinical signs in the Wernicke–Korsakoff complex: a retrospective analysis of 131 cases diagnosed at necropsy. *Journal of Neurology, Neurosurgery and Psychiatry.* **49**: 341–5.

20 Rees LH, Besser GM, Jeffcoate WJ *et al.* (1977) Alcohol-induced pseudo-Cushing's syndrome. *Lancet.* **i**: 726–8.

21 Beattie JO, Hull D and Cockburn F (1986) Children intoxicated by alcohol in Nottingham and Glasgow, 1973–84. *British Medical Journal.* **292**: 519–21.

22 Valimaki M and Ylikahri R (1983) The effect of alcohol on male and female sexual function. *Alcohol and Alcoholism.* **18**: 313–20.

23 Morgan MY (1982) The effects of moderate alcohol consumption on male fertility. In *The Endocrines and the Liver* (eds M Langer *et al.*), pp. 157–8. Academic Press, London.

24 Plant M (1992) Alcohol and breast cancer: a review. *International Journal of the Addictions.* **27**: 107–28.

25 Stratton K, Howe C and Battaglia F (eds) (1996) *Fetal Alcohol Syndrome. Diagnosis, Epidemiology, Prevention, and Treatment.* National Academy Press, Washington, DC.

26 Plant ML (1987) *Women, Drinking and Pregnancy* (2nd edn). Tavistock/Routledge, London.

27 Berti F, Rossoni G and Bella BD (1993) Bronchospasm during disulfiram–ethanol test reaction [letter]. *British Medical Journal.* **306**: 396.

28 Poikolainen K, Reunala T, Karvonen J *et al.* (1990) Alcohol intake: a risk factor for psoriasis in young and middle-aged men? *British Medical Journal.* **300**: 780–3.

29 Sacanella E, Fernandez-Solà J, Cofan M *et al* (1995) Chronic alcoholic myopathy: diagnostic clues and relationship with other alcohol-related diseases. *Quarterly Journal of Medicine.* **88**: 811–7.

30 Rico H (1990) Alcohol and bone disease. *Alcohol and Alcoholism.* **25**: 345–52.

31 Szabo G (1997) Alcohol's contribution to compromised immunity. *Alcohol Health and Research World.* **21**: 30–8.

Chapter 4: To learn more

Anderson P, Wallace P and Jones H (1988) *Alcohol Problems: practical problems for general practice 5.* Oxford University Press, Oxford.

Paton A (ed) (1994) *ABC of Alcohol* (3rd edn). BMJ Publishing, London.

Peters TJ and Edwards G (eds) (1994) *Alcohol and Alcohol Problems.* British Medical Bulletin, London.

Rix KJB (1983) *Alcohol Problems: a guide for nurses and other health professionals.* John Wright, Bristol.

Royal College of Physicians (1987) *A Great and Growing Evil: the medical consequences of alcohol abuse.* Tavistock, London.

Chapter 5

1 Oostveen T, Knibbe R and De Vries H (1996) Social influences on young adults' alcohol consumption: norms, modelling, pressure, socializing, and conformity. *Addict Behav.* **21**:187–97.

2 Room R (1994) Adolescent drinking as collective behavior and performance. In *The Development of Alcohol Problems: exploring the biopsychosocial matrix of risk* (eds R Zucker, G Boyd and J Howard). Research Monograph No. 26. NIH Publication No. 94-3495, National Institutes of Health.

3 Aitken PP (1985) Observational study of young adults' drinking groups. II. Drink purchasing procedures, group pressures and alcohol consumption by companions as predictors of alcohol consumption. *Alcohol and Alcoholism*. **20**: 445–57.

4 Power C and Estaugh V (1990) Role of family formation and dissolution in shaping drinking behaviour in early adulthood. *Br J Addict*. **85**: 521–30.

5 Neve R (1998) The Life Course, Gender, and Alcohol Use. Thesis, Maastricht.

6 Hammer T and Vaglum P (1990) Use of alcohol and drugs in the transitional phase from adolescence to young adulthood. *J Adolesc*. **13**: 129–42.

7 Parker DA and Harford TC (1992) Gender-role attitudes, job competition and alcohol consumption among women and men. *Alcohol Clin Exp Res*. **16**: 159–65.

8 Ahlström-Laakso S (1976) European drinking habits: a review of research and some suggestions for conceptual integration of findings. In *Cross-Cultural Approaches to the Study of Alcohol: an interdisciplinary perspective* (eds MW Everett, JO Waddell and DB Heath). Mouton Publishers, The Hague, Paris.

9 Hibell B, Andersson B, Bjarnason T *et al.* (eds) (1997) *The 1995 ESPAD Report. Alcohol and Other Drug Use Among Students in 26 European Countries*. Modin Tryck AB, Stockholm.

10 Nahoum-Grappe V (1995) France. In *International Handbook on Alcohol and Culture* (ed DB Heath). Greenwood Press, Westport, Connecticut, London.

11 Miller H, Turner C and Moses L (eds) (1990) *AIDS: the second decade*. National Academy Press, Washington, DC.

12 Ahlström S, Haavisto K, Tuovinen EL *et al.* (1997) Finnish Country Report for the European School Survey Project on Alcohol and Drugs (ESPAD), *Themes No1/1997. STAKES*, Helsinki.

13 Plant M and Plant M (1992) *Risk-Takers: alcohol, drugs, sex and youth*. Tavistock/Routledge, London.

14 Parker DA, Harford TC and Rosenstock IM (1994) Alcohol, other drugs, and sexual risk-taking among young adults. *J Subst Abuse*. **6**: 87–93.

15 Miller P, Plant M, Plant M *et al.* (1995) Alcohol, tobacco, illicit drugs, and sex: an analysis of risky behaviours among young adults. *Int J Addict*. **30**: 239–58.

Chapter 5: To learn more

Edwards G, Anderson P, Babor TF *et al.* (1994) *Alcohol Policy and the Public Good*. Oxford University Press, Oxford.

Gottfredson DC, Gottfredson GD and Skroban S (1998) Can prevention work when it is needed most? *Evaluation Review*. **22**: 315–39.

Hannibal JU, van Iwaarden MJ, Gefou-Madianou D *et al.* (1995) *Alcohol and the Community*. World Health Organization Regional Office for Europe, Salomon & Roussell A/S, Denmark.

Holder H and Howard JM (eds) (1992) *Community Prevention Trials for Alcohol Problems: methodological issues*. Praeger Publishers, Westport.

Holmila M (ed) (1997) *Community Prevention of Alcohol Problems*. Macmillan Press Ltd, London.

Home Office (1998) *Drug Misuse and the Environment. A report by the Advisory Council on the Misuse of Drugs*, The Stationery Office, London.

Plant M, Single E and Stockwell T (eds) (1997) *Alcohol: minimising the harm. What works?* Free Association Books Ltd, London.

Chapter 6

Except where references refer to specific studies, they will tend to be representative of the view expressed. They have been chosen in part to provide further useful sources of information.

1 Barr A (1995) *Drink: an informal social history*. Bantam Press, London.

2 Ibid.

3 Powers M (1995) Women and public drinking, 1890–1920. *History Today*. **52** (Feb): 46–53.

4 Banwell C (1991) I'm not a drinker really: women and alcohol. In *Ladies a Plate* (ed J Park). Auckland University Press, Auckland.

5 Smith R (1991) Who am I? Identity. In *Ladies a Plate* (ed J Park). Auckland University Press, Auckland.

6 Heath DB (1995) *Handbook on Alcohol and Culture*. Greenwood International Press, Connecticut.

7 Popkin CL (1991) Drinking and driving by young females. *Accident Analysis and Prevention*. **23**(1): 37–44.

8 Wilsnack SC and Wilsnack R (1995) Drinking and problem drinking in US women. In *Recent Developments in Alcoholism, Vol. 12: Women and Alcoholism* (ed M Galanter), pp. 29–60. Plenum Press, New York.

9 Wilsnack SC and Wilsnack RW (1993) Epidemiological research on women's drinking: recent progress and directions for the 1990s. In *Women and Substance Abuse* (eds ESL Gomberg and TD Nirenberg). Ablex Publishing, Norwood, NJ.

10 Nunes-Dinis MC and Weisner C (1997) Gender differences in the relationship of alcohol and drug use to criminal behavior in a sample of arrestees. *American Journal of Drug and Alcohol Abuse*. **23**(1): 129–41.

11 Wilsnack SC, Wilsnack RW and Hiller-Sturmhofel S (1994) How women drink: epidemiology of women's drinking and problem drinking. *Alcohol Health and Research World*. **18**(3): 173–81.

12 Wyllie A, Millard M and Zhang JF (1996) *Drinking in New Zealand*. University of Auckland, Auckland.

13 Goddard E (1997) *Drinking: adults' behaviour and knowledge*. Office for National Statistics, Social Survey Division, London.

14 Yu J and Perrine W (1997) The transmission of parent/child drinking patterns: testing a gender-specific structural model. *American Journal of Drug and Alcohol Abuse*. **23**(1): 143–65.

15 Kunz J and Graham K (1996) Life course changes in alcohol consumption in leisure activities of men and women. *Journal of Drug Issues*. **26**(4): 805–29.

16 Duckert F (1996) Alcohol problems and recruitment to treatment. *Alcoholpolitic*. **8**(1): 30–8.

17 Miller WR and Cervantes EA (1997) Gender and patterns of alcohol problems: pretreatment responses of women and men to the comprehensive drinker profile. *Journal of Clinical Psychology.* **53**(3): 263–77.

18 Snow MG, Prochaska JO and Rossi JS (1994) Processes of change in Alcoholics Anonymous: maintenance factors in long-term sobriety. *Journal of Studies on Alcohol.* **55**: 362–71.

19 Dawson D (1996) Gender differences in the risk of alcohol dependence. *Addiction.* **91**(12): 1831–42.

20 Plant M (1997) *Women and Alcohol*, p. 70. Free Association Books, London.

21 Ibid.

22 Ibid. pp. 24, 25.

23 Ibid. pp. 89–93, 96–8.

24 Sampson P, Streissguth A, Bookstein F *et al.* (1997) Incidence of fetal alcohol syndrome and prevalence of alcohol-related neurodevelopmental disorder. *Teratology.* **56**: 317–26.

25 MacEwan I (1997) *Treatment differences in outcome between females and males.* In *Cutting Edge '97.* Proceedings of the Annual National Treatment Conference. Alcohol Advisory Council of New Zealand, Wellington.

26 Ibid.

27 McCallum T (1998) *Gender differences in youth drug use.* Australian Conference: Addictions: Challenges and Changes. Research presentation.

28 Ibid.

29 Wyllie A and Casswell S (1991) A qualitative investigation of young men's drinking in New Zealand. *Health Education Research: Theory and Practice.* **6**(1): 49–55.

30 Archer A (1990) Maori and European attitudes, motivations and practices toward alcohol consumption with specific reference to drinking and driving. University of Canterbury dissertation.

31 Casswell S, Stewart J, Connolly G *et al.* (1991) A longitudinal study of New Zealand children's experience with alcohol. *British Journal of Addiction.* **86**: 277–85.

32 Plant M (1997) *Women and Alcohol.* Free Association Books, London.

33 Ibid.

34 Ibid.

35 Pearce EJ and Lovejoy FH (1995) Detecting a history of childhood sexual experiences among women substance-abusers. *Journal of Substance Abuse Treatment.* **12**(4): 283–7.

36 Vannicelli M (1992) *Removing the Roadblocks.* Guilford Press, New York.

37 Toneatto A, Sobell LC and Sobell MB (1992) Gender issues in the treatment of abusers of alcohol, nicotine, and other drugs. *Journal of Substance Abuse.* **4**: 209–18.

38 Rubin A, Stout R and Longabaugh R (1996) Gender differences in relapse situations. *Addiction.* **91**: 111–20.

39 Wilsnack RW and Wright SI (1991) *Women in predominantly male occupations: relationships to problem drinking.* Paper presented at the Annual Meeting of the Society for the Study of Social Problems, Cincinnati, OH.

40 Ibid.
41 Klassen AD (1996) Sexual experience and drinking among women in a national survey. *Alcohol Health and Research World*. **20**(4): 181–92.

Chapter 6: To learn more

Barr A (1995) *Drink: an informal social history*. Bantam Press, London.
Heath DB (1995) *Handbook on Alcohol and Culture*. Greenwood International Press, Connecticut.
Plant M (1997) *Women and Alcohol*. Free Association Books, London.
Vannicelli M (1992) *Removing the Roadblocks*. Guilford Press, New York.

Chapter 7

1 Faculty of Public Health Medicine (1991) *Alcohol and the Public Health*. MacMillan, London.
2 Collins R, Leonard K and Searles J (eds) (1990) *Alcohol and the Family*. Guilford Press, New York.
3 Velleman R (1993) *Alcohol and the Family*. Institute of Alcohol Studies Occasional Paper. Institute of Alcohol Studies, London.
4 Rutter M (1980) *Maternal Deprivation Reassessed* (2nd edn). Penguin, London.
5 Velleman R and Orford J (1999) *Risk and Resilience: adults who were the children of problem drinkers*. Harwood, London.
6 Meyer M (1982) *Drinking Problems Equal Family Problems: practical guidelines for the problem drinker, the partner and all those involved*. Momenta, Lancaster.
7 Seixas J (1980) *How to Cope with an Alcoholic Parent*. Canongate, Edinburgh.

Chapter 7: To learn more

Collins R, Leonard K and Searles J (eds) (1990) *Alcohol and the Family*. Guilford Press, New York.
Meyer M (1982) *Drinking Problems Equal Family Problems: practical guidelines for the problem drinker, the partner and all those involved*. Momenta, Lancaster.
Orford J (ed) (1986) *Coping with Disorder in the Family*. Croom Helm, London.
Paolino T and McCrady B (1978) *Marriage and Marital Therapy*. Bruner/Mazel, New York.
Seixas J (1980) *How to Cope with an Alcoholic Parent*. Canongate, Edinburgh.
Stanton M and Todd T (1982) *The Family Therapy of Drug Abuse and Addiction*. Guilford Press, New York.
Velleman R, Copello A and Maslin J (eds) (1998) *Living With Drink: women who live with problem drinkers*. Longman, London.
Velleman R and Orford J (1999) *Risk and Resilience: adults who were the children of problem drinkers*. Harwood, London.

Chapter 8

1 Douglas M (1991) *Constructive Drinking: perspectives on drinking from anthropology*. Cambridge University Press, Cambridge.
2 Scott RB (1989) Alcohol effects in the elderly. *Comparative Therapies*. **15**: 8–12.
3 Blazer D, George L, Woodbury M *et al.* (1984) The elderly alcoholic: a profile. In *Nature and Extent of Alcohol Problems Among the Elderly* (eds G Madox, LN Robins and N Rosenberg). NIAAA Research Monograph No. 14, Rockville, Maryland.
4 Rosin AJ and Glatt MM (1971) Alcohol excess in the elderly. *Quarterly Journal of Studies on Alcohol*. **32**: 53–9.
5 Graham K, Zeidman A, Flower MC *et al.* (1992) A typology of elderly persons with alcohol problems. *Alcoholism Treatment Quarterly*. **9**(3/4): 79–95.
6 Kane R and Kane R (1981) *Assessing the Elderly: a practical guide to measurement*. Lexington Books, Lexington, Massachusetts.
7 Oliver R, Blathwayt J, Brackley C *et al.* (1993) Development of the Safety Assessment of Function and the Environment for Rehabilitation (SAFER) Tool. *Canadian J Occupational Therapy*. **60**(2): 78–82.
8 Hinrichsen JJ (1984) Toward improving treatment services for alcoholics of advanced age. *Alcohol Health and Research World*. **8**(3): 31–9.
9 Graham K (1986) Identifying and measuring alcohol abuse among the elderly: serious problems with existing instrumentation. *Journal of Studies on Alcohol*. **47**(4): 322–6.
10 American Medical Association Council on Scientific Affairs (1996) Alcoholism in the elderly. *Journal of the American Medical Association*. **275**(10): 797–801.
11 LESA (Lifestyles Enrichment for Senior Adults Program), ARF (Addiction Research Foundation) and COPA (Community Older Persons Alcohol Program) (1993) *Alternatives: prevention and intervention for alcohol and drug problems in seniors*. ARF, Toronto.
12 Blow FC (1992*) Michigan Alcoholism Screening Test – Geriatric Version (MAST-G): a new elderly-specific screening instrument*. Presented at the 38th Annual Meeting of the American Society on Aging, March 15, 1992, San Diego, California.
13 COPA (Community Older Persons Alcohol Program) (1998) Material developed for educational and instructive purposes. See pp. 256–7 for contact information.
14 Gurnack A (ed) (1997) *Older Adults' Misuse of Alcohol, Medicines and Other Drugs: research and practice issues*. Springer Press, New York.
15 Saunders SJ, Graham K, Flower MC *et al.* (1992) The COPA Project as a model for the management of early dementia in the community. In *Care-giving in Dementia* (eds GMM Jones and BML Miesen). Tavistock/Routledge, New York.
16 Miller WR and Rollnick S (1991) *Motivational Interviewing: preparing people to change addictive behavior*, p. xi. Guilford Press, New York.
17 Ibid, p. 192.
18 Addictions Foundation of Manitoba. Brochure titled *Gambling and Seniors: prevention and recognition of problem gambling*. Winnipeg, Manitoba.
19 Cooper DB (1994) *Alcohol Home Detoxification and Assessment*. Radcliffe Medical Press, Oxford.
20 Stockwell T (1987) The Exeter Home Detoxification Project. In: *Helping the Problem Drinker: a new initiative in community care* (eds T Stockwell and S Clement). Croom Helm, London.

21 McKee E (1997) *There's No Place Like Home*. Report available at the COPA Program. (See below for contact information.)

22 Steinmetz SK (1990) Elder abuse: myth and reality. In *Family Relations in Later Life* (ed TH Brubaker), p. 209. SAGE Publications, Newbury Park, California.

23 Addictions Treatment Programs and the Older Adult – Evaluation. In progress. Contact COPA Program. (See below for contact information.)

24 Evaluation of Phase I of COPA Telephone Consultation Service (1998). Available by contacting the author at COPA. (See below for contact information.)

Chapter 8: To learn more

Alternatives: prevention and intervention for alcohol and drug problems in seniors. LESA (Lifestyles Enrichment for Senior Adults Program), ARF (Addiction Research Foundation) and COPA (Community Older Persons Alcohol Program) (1993) ARF, Toronto. Cost $150.00 Canadian. To order, call:

Center for Addiction and Mental Health Marketing Services
33 Russell St
Toronto
M5S 2S1
Canada
Telephone from Continental North America: 1- (800) 661 1111
From other locations: (416) 535 8501
Fax number: (416) 593 4694
E-mail: mktg@arf.org

Choosing to Change. Handbook in development. Introducing home-visiting professionals to identification and engagement skills that are relevant to older adults with substance use problems. For information call:

Center for Addiction and Mental Health Marketing Services
33 Russell St
Toronto
M5S 2S1
Canada
Telephone from Continental North America: 1- (800) 661 1111
From other locations: (416) 535 8501
Fax number: (416) 593 4694
E-mail: mktg@arf.org

For information about the Addictions Service's Organizational Sensitizing Questionnaire or Standards of Care – Requirements and Qualifications, contact the author at:

COPA
27 Roncesvalles Ave., Suite 407
Toronto
M6R 3B2
Canada
Telephone: (416) 516 2982
Fax: (416) 516 2984
E-mail: copa@interlog.com

Dupree LW, Broslowski H and Schonfeld L (1984) The Gerontology Alcohol Project: a behavioral treatment program for elderly alcohol abusers. *Gerontologist.* **24**(5): 510–16.

Chapter 9

1 McDermott F and Pyett P (1993) *Not Welcome Anywhere.* Victorian Community-Managed Mental Health Services, Inc., Melbourne.
2 Early Psychosis Prevention and Intervention Centre (1997) Information Sheet No. 1. EPPIC Statewide Services, Victoria.
3 Sumich HJ, Andrews G and Hunt CJ (1995) *The Management of Mental Disorders.* World Health Organization, Sydney, Australia.
4 Ananth J, Vanewater S, Kanal M *et al.* (1989) Missed diagnosis of substance abuse in psychiatric patients. *Hospital and Community Psychiatry.* **40**(3): 297–9.
5 Fox T, Fox L and Drake RE (1992) *Developing a stateside service system for people with co-occurring mental illness and substance disorders.* [Unpublished.] Dartmouth Psychiatric Research Center, New Hampshire.
6 Drake RE, Antosca L, Noordsy DL *et al.* (1992) New Hampshire's specialized services for people dually diagnosed with severe mental illness and substance use disorder. *New Directions for Mental Health Services.* **50**: 57–67.
7 Ries RK and Ellingson T (1990) A pilot assessment at one month of 17 dual diagnosis patients. *Hospital and Community Psychiatry.* **41**(11): 1230–3.
8 Salloum IM, Moss HB and Daley DC (1991) Substance abuse and schizophrenia: impediments to optimal care. *American Journal of Drug and Alcohol Abuse.* **17**(3): 321–36.
9 Regier DA, Myers JK, Kramer M *et al.* (1984) The NIMH Epidemiolgic Catchment Area Program: historical context, major objectives, and study population characteristics. *Archives of General Psychiatry.* **41**: 934–41.
10 Christie KA, Burke JD, Reiger DA *et al.* (1988) Epidemiological evidence for early onset of mental disorders and high risk of drug abuse in young adults. *American Journal of Psychiatry.* **148**(8): 771–5.
11 Bergman HC and Harris M (1985) Substance abuse among young-adult chronic patients. *Psychosocial Rehabilitation Journal.* **9**(1): 49–54.
12 Dixon L, Gretchen H, Weidon PJ *et al.* (1991). Drug abuse in schizophrenia patients: clinical correlates and reasons for use. *American Journal of Psychiatry.* **148**(2): 224–30.

13 Noordsy DL (1991) Subjective experience related to alcohol use among schizophrenics. *Journal of Nervous and Mental Disorders.* **179**: 410–14.

14 Barbee JG, Clark PO, Cropanzane MS *et al.* (1989) Alcohol and substance abuse among schizophrenic patients presenting to an emergency psychiatric service. *Journal of Nervous and Mental Disorders.* **177**: 400–7.

15 Carey KB, Carey MP and Meister AW (1991) Psychiatric symptoms in mentally ill chemical abusers. *Journal of Nervous and Mental Disorders.* **179**(3): 136–8.

16 Mueser KT, Yarnold PR, Levinson DK *et al.* (1990) Prevalence of substance abuse in schizophrenia. Demographic and clinical correlates. *Schizophrenia Bulletin.* **16**: 31–56.

17 Drake RE, Osher FC and Wallach MA (1989) Alcohol use and abuse in schizophrenia: a perspective community study. *Journal of Nervous and Mental Disorders.* **177**: 408–14.

18 Yesavage JA and Zarcone V (1983) History of drug abuse and dangerous behaviour in inpatient schizophrenics. *Journal of Clinical Psychiatry.* **44**: 259–61.

19 Alterman AL, Erdlen FR, McLelland AT *et al.* (1980) Problem drinking in hospitalised schizophrenic patients. *Addictive Behaviours.* **5**: 273–6.

20 Hayward L, Zubrick SR and Silburn S (1992) Blood alcohol levels in suicide cases. *Journal of Epidemiology and Community Health.* **46**: 256–60.

21 Rich CL, Fowler RC, Fogarty LA *et al.* (1998) San Diego suicide study III. Relationships between diagnoses and stressors. *Archives of General Psychiatry.* **45**: 589–92.

22 Beautrais AL, Joyce PR, Mulder RT *et al.* (1996) Prevalence and comorbidity of mental disorders in persons making serious suicide attempts: a case–control study. *American Journal of Psychiatry.* **153**(8): 1009–14.

Chapter 9: To learn more

McDermott F and Pyett P (1993) *Not Welcome Anywhere*. Victorian Community-Managed Mental Health Services, Inc., Melbourne.

Sumich HJ, Andrews G and Hunt CJ (1995) *The Management of Mental Disorders*. World Health Organization, Sydney, Australia.

Chapter 10

1 Linton R (1947) *The Study of Man*. Appleton, New York.

2 Brown C (1963) *Understanding Other Cultures*, p. 11. Prentice-Hall, Englewood Cliffs, NJ.

3 Orlandi MA (1992) The challenge of evaluating community-based prevention programs: a cross-cultural perspective. In *Cultural Competence for Evaluators: a guide for alcohol and other drug abuse prevention practitioners working with ethnic/racial communities*, pp. 1–22. Office for Substance Abuse Prevention, US Dept of Health and Human Service, Rockville, MD.

4 Gray D and Morfitt B (1996) Harm minimisation in an indigenous context. In *Cultural variations in the meaning of harm minimisation: their implications for policy*

and practice in the drugs arena, pp. 53–63. Proceedings of a regional conference convened by the WHO Collaborating Centre for Prevention and Control of Alcohol and Drug Abuse, Perth, Australia.

5 Degrassi S and Inge L (1997) *Cultural Diversity – An Overview of the Issues*. Cultural Diversity Training Unit, University of Sydney, Australia.

6 French L (1989) Theory and practice, Native American alcoholism: a transcultural counselling perspective. *Counselling Psychology Quarterly*. **2**(2): 153–66.

7 Tannen D (1991) *You Just Don't Understand: women and men in conversation*, pp. 201–2. Random House, Australia.

8 Walsh D, Cook JP, Davis K *et al*. *The cultural dimensions of alcohol policy worldwide*. International Symposium on the Cultural Dimensions of Alcohol Policy Worldwide. Salzburg Seminars, Health Affairs, Summer 1989.

9 Heath DB (1991) Women and alcohol: cross-cultural perspectives. *Journal of Substance Abuse*. **3**: 175–85.

10 Young K (1995) *Alcohol misuse and violence: cross-cultural analysis of the relationship between alcohol and violence*. Report 3. National Symposium on Alcohol Misuse and Violence. Drug Offensive, Australia.

Chapter 10: To learn more

Adlaf EM, Smart RG and Tan SH (1989) Ethnicity and drug use: a critical look. *International Journal of the Addictions*. **24**: 1–18.

Anglin DM, Ryan TM, Booth MW *et al*. (1988) Ethnic differences in narcotic addiction: characteristics of Chicano and Anglo methadone maintenance clients. *International Journal of the Addictions*. **23**: 125–49.

Austin GA, Johnson BD, Carroll EE *et al*. (1987) *Drugs and Minorities*. Research Issues 21. DBEW publication No. (ADM) 78-507. NIDA, Rockville, MD.

Barbor TF (ed) (1986) Alcohol and culture: comparative perspectives from Europe and America. *Annals of the New York Academy of Sciences*. **472**.

Bennett LA and Ames GM (ed) (1955) *The American Experience with Alcohol: contrasting cultural perspectives*. Plenum Press, New York.

Bounds M (1980) Cultural perspectives on social drug use. In *Man, drugs and society: current perspectives*. Proceedings of the first Pan-Pacific Conference on Drugs and Alcohol. Australian Foundation on Alcoholism and Drug Dependence, Canberra, Australia.

Chapter 11

1 Rorabaugh WJ (1979) *The Alcoholic Republic and American Tradition*. Oxford University Press, New York.

2 Jernigan D (1997) *Thirsting for Markets: the global impact of corporate alcohol*. The Marin Institute for the Prevention of Alcohol and Other Drug Problems, San Rafael, CA.

3 Fillmore K and Caetano R (1982) Epidemiology of alcohol abuse and alcoholism in occupations. In *Occupational Alcoholism: a review of research issues*. NIAAA Research Monograph No. 8. US Government Printing Office, Washington, DC.

4 Trice HM and Sonnenstuhl WJ (1990) On the construction of drinking norms in work organizations. *Journal of Studies on Alcohol*. **51**: 201–20.

5 Parker DA and Harford TC (1992) The epidemiology of alcohol consumption and dependence across occupations in the United States. *Alcohol Health and Research World*. **16**: 97–105.

6 Mandell W, Eaton WW, Anthony JC *et al.* (1992) Alcoholism and occupations: a review and analysis of 104 occupations. *Alcoholism: Clinical and Experimental Research*. **16**: 306–17.

7 Ames GM and Janes CR (1992) A cultural approach to conceptualizing alcohol and the workplace. *Alcohol Health and Research World*. **16**: 112–19.

8 Janes CR and Ames GM (1993) The workplace. In *Recent Developments in Alcoholism, Volume 11: Ten Years of Progress* (ed M Galanter). Plenum Press, New York.

9 Delaney WP and Ames GM (1995) Work team attitudes, drinking norms, and workplace drinking. *Journal of Drug Issues*. **25**: 275–90.

10 Sonnenstuhl WJ and Trice HM (1987) The social construction of alcohol problems in a union's peer counseling program. *Journal of Drug Issues*. **17**: 223–54.

11 Sonnenstuhl WJ (1996) *Working Sober: transformation of an occupational drinking culture*. ILR Press, Ithaca, NY.

12 Howland J, Mangione TW, Kuhlthau K *et al.* (1996) Work-site variation in managerial drinking. *Addiction*. **91**: 1007–17.

13 Roman PM, Blum TC and Martin JK (1992) 'Enabling' of male problem drinkers in work groups. *British Journal of Addiction*. **87**: 275–89.

14 Manello TA and Seaman FJ (1979) *Prevalence, Costs and Handling of Drinking Problems at Seven Railroads*. University Research Corporation, Washington, DC.

15 Ames GM and Janes CR (1987) Heavy and problem drinking in an American blue-collar population. *Social Science Medicine*. **25**: 949–60.

16 Conway T, Vickers R, Ward H *et al.* (1981) Occupational stress and variation in cigarette, coffee, and alcohol consumption. *Journal of Health and Social Behavior*. **22**: 155–65.

17 Parker D and Farmer G (1990) Employed adults at risk for diminished self-control over alcohol use: the alienated, the burned out, and the unchallenged. In *Alcohol Problem Intervention in the Workplace: employee assistance programs and strategic alternatives*. (ed PM Roman). Quorum Books, Westport, CT.

18 Martin JK, Blum TC and Roman PM (1992) Drinking to cope and self-medication: characteristics of jobs in relation to workers' drinking behavior. *Journal of Organizational Behavior*. **13**: 55–71.

19 Martin JK, Roman PM and Blum TC (1996) Job stress, drinking networks, and social support at work: a comprehensive model of employees' problem drinking behaviors. *Sociological Quarterly*. **37**: 201–21.

20 Kohn M and Schooler C (1973) Occupational experience and psychological functioning: an assessment of reciprocal effects. *American Sociological Review*. **38**: 97–118.

21 Fennell ML, Rodin MB and Kantor GK (1981) Problems in the work setting: drinking and reasons for drinking. *Social Forces*. **60**: 114–32.

22 Kavanaugh MJ, Hurst M and Rose R (1981) The relationship between job satisfaction and psychiatric health symptoms for air traffic controllers. *Personnel Psychology*. **34**: 691–707.

23 Karasek R, Gardell G and Lindell J (1987) Work and non-work correlates of illness and behavior in male and female Swedish white-collar workers. *Journal of Occupational Behavior*. **8**: 187–207.

24 Harris M and Fennell ML (1988) A multivariate model of job stress and alcohol consumption. *Sociological Quarterly*. **29**: 391–406.

25 Janes CR and Ames GM (1989) Men, blue-collar work and drinking: alcohol use in an industrial subculture. *Culture, Medicine and Psychiatry*. **13**: 245–74.

26 Cooper ML, Russell M and Frone MR (1990) Work stress and alcohol effects: a test of stress-induced drinking. *Journal of Health and Social Behavior*. **31**: 260–76.

27 Richman JA (1992) Occupational stress, psychological vulnerability and alcohol-related problems over time in future physicians. *Alcoholism: Clinical and Experimental Research*. **16**: 166–71.

28 Richman JA, Flaherty JA and Rospenda KM (1996) Perceived workplace harassment experiences and problem drinking among physicians. *Addiction*. **91**: 391–403.

29 Hammer T and Vaglum P (1989) The increase in alcohol consumption among women: a phenomenon related to accessibility or stress? A general population study. *British Journal of Addiction*. **84**: 767–75.

30 Shore ER (1990) Business and professional women: primary prevention for new role incumbents. In *Alcohol Problem Intervention in the Workplace: employee assistance programs and strategic alternatives* (ed PM Roman). Quorum Books, Westport, CT.

31 Wilsnack RW and Wilsnack SC (1992) Women, work, and alcohol: failures of simple theories. *Alcoholism: Clinical and Experimental Research*. **16**: 172–9.

32 Shore ER (1992) Drinking patterns and problems among women in paid employment. *Alcohol, Health and Research World*. **16**: 160–4.

33 Parker DA, Parker ES, Wolz MW *et al.* (1980) Sex roles and alcohol consumption: a research note. *Journal of Health and Social Behavior*. **21**: 43–8.

34 Steinberg L, Fegley S and Dornbusch SM (1993) Negative impact of part-time work on adolescent adjustment: evidence from a longitudinal study. *Developmental Psychology*. **29**: 171–80.

35 Steinberg L and Dornbusch SM (1991) Negative correlates of part-time employment during adolescence: replication and elaboration. *Developmental Psychology*. **27**: 304–13.

36 Roman PM and Johnson JA (1996) Alcohol's role in workforce entry and retirement. *Alcohol, Health and Research World*. **20**: 162–9.

37 Sanford M, Offord D, McLeod K *et al.* (1994) Pathways into the workforce: antecedents of school and workforce status. *Journal of the American Academy of Child and Adolescent Psychiatry*. **33**: 1036–46.

38 Mullahy J and Sindelar JL (1989) Life-cycle effect of alcoholism on education, earnings, and occupation. *Inquiry*. **26**: 272–82.

39 Mullahy J and Sindelar JL (1991) Gender differences in labor market effects of alcoholism. *American Economic Review*. **81**: 161–5.

40 Vaillant GE (1995) *The Natural History of Alcoholism Revisited.* Harvard University Press, Cambridge, MA.

41 Mirand AL and Welte JW (1996) Alcohol consumption among the elderly in a general population, Erie County, New York. *American Journal of Public Health.* **86**: 978–84.

42 Mertens JR, Moos RH and Brennan PL (1996) Alcohol consumption, life context, and coping predict mortality among late-middle-aged drinkers and former drinkers. *Alcoholism: Clinical and Experimental Research.* **20**: 313–19.

43 Ekerdt DJ, De Labry LO, Glynn RJ *et al.* (1989) Change in drinking behaviors with retirement: findings from the Normative Aging Study. *Journal of Studies on Alcohol.* **50**: 347–53.

44 Finney JW and Moos RH (1984) Life stressors and problem drinking among older adults. In *Recent Developments in Alcoholism*, Vol. 2 (ed M Galanter). Plenum Press, New York.

45 Cahalan D and Cisin IH (1968) American drinking practices: summary of findings from a national probability sample. *Quarterly Journal of Studies on Alcohol.* **29**: 130–51.

46 Barnes GM (1979) Alcohol use among older persons: findings from a western New York State general population survey. *Journal of the American Geriatrics Society.* **27**: 244–50.

47 Gurnack AM and Thomas JL (1989) Behavioral factors related to elderly alcohol abuse: research and policy issues. *International Journal of the Addictions.* **24**: 641–54.

48 Gurnack AM and Hoffman NG (1992) Elderly alcohol misuse. *International Journal of the Addictions.* **27**: 869–78.

Chapter 11: To learn more

Denenberg TS and Denenberg RV (1983) *Alcohol and Drugs: issues in the workplace.* Bureau of National Affairs, Washington, DC.

Hore BD and Plant MA (eds) (1981) *Alcohol Problems in Employment.* Croom Helm, London.

Normand J, Lempert RO and O'Brien CP (1994) *Under the Influence: drugs and the American workforce.* National Academy Press, Washington, DC.

Roman PM (1990) *Alcohol Problem Intervention in the Workplace: employee assistance programs and strategic alternatives.* Quorum Books, New York.

Sonnenstuhl WJ (1996) *Working Sober: transformation of an occupational drinking culture.* ILR Press, Ithaca, NY.

Trice HM and Roman PM (1978) *Spirits and Demons at Work: alcohol and other drugs on the job.* ILR Press, Ithaca, NY.

Chapter 12

1 Roberts C (1996) The physiological effects of alcohol misuse. *Professional Nurse.* **11**(10): 646–8.

2 Edwards G, Anderson P and Babor TF (1994) *Alcohol Policy and the Public Good.* Oxford University Press, Oxford.

3 Hartz C, Plant M and Watt M (1990) *Alcohol and Health: a handbook for nurses, midwives and health visitors.* The Medical Council on Alcoholism, London.

4 Godfrey C (1996) The economic impact of alcohol misuse and abuse. In *Alcohol Dependency: meeting the challenge.* Tangent Medical Education, London.

5 Lehto J (1997) The economics of alcohol. *Addiction.* **92**(1): S55–S59.

6 Skinner HA and Holt S (1983) Early intervention for alcohol problems. *Journal of the Royal College of General Practitioners.* **33**: 787–91.

7 Saunders JB and Aasland OG (1987) *WHO Collaborative Project on Identification and Treatment of Persons with Harmful Alcohol Consumption. Report on phase 1: development of an instrument.* World Health Organization, Division of Mental Health, Geneva.

8 Institute of Medicine (1990) *Broadening the Base of Treatment for Alcohol Problems.* National Academy Press, Washington, DC.

9 Heather N (1996) The public health and brief interventions for excessive alcohol consumption: the British experience. *Addictive Behaviours.* **21**(6): 857–68.

10 World Health Organization (1978) *The Declaration at Alma Ata: Health for All Series 1.* WHO, Geneva.

11 Kreitman N (1986) Alcohol consumption and the preventive paradox. *British Journal of Addiction.* **81**: 353–63.

12 Rose J (1992) *The Strategy of Preventative Medicine.* Oxford University Press, Oxford.

13 Royal College of General Practitioners (1986) *Alcohol: a balanced view.* RCGP, London.

14 Royal College of Physicians (1987) *A Great and Growing Evil: the medical consequences of alcohol abuse.* Tavistock, London.

15 British Medical Association (1995) *Alcohol: guidelines for sensible drinking.* BMA, London.

16 Duffy JC (ed) (1992) *Alcohol and Illness: the epidemiological viewpoint.* Edinburgh University Press, Edinburgh.

17 Marmott MG, Elliott P and Shiplet MJ (1994) Alcohol and blood pressure: the INTERSALT study. *British Medical Journal.* **308**: 1263–7.

18 Downie RS, Tannahill C and Tannahill A (1996) *Health Promotion: models and values* (2nd edn), p. 25. Oxford University Press, Oxford.

19 Sheffield Health Promotion (1996). Cited in McCulloch GF and Boxer J (1997) *Mental Health Promotion: policy practice and partnerships,* p. 9. Bailliere Tindall, London.

20 Armstrong EM and Robins SAC (1996) Prevention of alcohol-related harm. *Journal of Substance Misuse.* **1**(4): 195–8.

21 Godfrey C (1997). Cited in Plant M, Single E and Stockwell T (eds) (1997) *Alcohol: minimising the harm,* Ch 3. Free Association Books, London.

22 National Highway Traffic Safety Administration (1990; 1995). Cited in Plant M, Single E and Stockwell T (eds) (1997) *Alcohol: minimising the harm*, p. 17, 18. Free Association Books, London.

23 Robson WJ (1998) Alcohol and adolescents. *Journal of Substance Misuse*. 3(1): 3–4.

24 Gusfield J (1986). Cited in Plant M, Single E and Stockwell T (eds) (1997) *Alcohol: minimising the harm*, Ch 2. Free Association Books, London.

25 Bennett P and Murphy S (1997) *Psychology and Health Promotion*, p. 92. Open University Press, Buckingham.

26 Duffy JC (1992) Scottish licensing reforms. In *Alcohol and Drugs: the Scottish experience* (eds M Plant, B Ritson and R Robertson). Edinburgh University Press, Edinburgh.

27 Stockwell T and Single E (1997) Standard unit labelling of alcohol containers. In *Alcohol: minimising the harm* (eds M Plant, E Single and T Stockwell). Free Association Books, London.

28 Deaver EL (1997) History and implications of Alcoholic Beverages Labelling Act, 1988. *Journal of Substance Misuse*. 2(4): 234–7.

29 Rix KJB and Rix EML (1983) *Alcohol Problems. A guide for nurses and other health professionals*, p. 158. Wright and Sons, London.

30 Bien TH, Miller WR and Tonigan JS (1993) Brief interventions for alcohol problems: a review. *Addiction*. **88**: 315–36.

31 Babor TF and Grant M (eds) (1992) *Project on Identification and Management of Alcohol-related Problems. Report on phase II: a randomized clinical trial of brief interventions in primary health care*. World Health Organization, Division of Mental Health, Geneva.

32 Holder H, Longabaugh R, Miller WR *et al.* (1991) The cost-effectiveness of treatment for alcoholism: a first approximation. *Journal of Studies on Alcohol*. **52**(6): 517–40.

33 Elvy GA, Wells JE and Baird KA (1988) Attempted referral as intervention for problem drinking in the general hospital. *British Journal of Addiction*. **83**: 83–9.

34 Chick J, Lloyd G and Crombie E (1985) Counselling problem drinkers in medical wards: a controlled study. *British Medical Journal*. **290**: 965–7.

35 Cooper DB (1993) Education on the rocks. *Nursing Times*. **89**(29): 32–6.

36 McBrien M (1983) The potential role of the nurse in prevention and early intervention in alcohol misuse. *Health Bulletin*. **41**(1): 23–5.

37 Anderson P, Wallace P and Jones H (1988) *Alcohol Problems – A Practical Guide for General Practice*. Oxford University Press, Oxford.

38 Murray A (1992) Minimal intervention with problem drinkers. In *Alcohol and Drugs: the Scottish experience* (eds M Plant, B Ritson and R Robertson). Edinburgh University Press, Edinburgh.

39 Duffy JC and Waterton JJ (1984) Under-reporting of alcohol consumption in sample surveys. *British Journal of Addiction*. **79**: 303–8.

40 Poikolainen K, Karkkainen P and Pikkarainen P (1985) Correlations between biological markers and alcohol intake, as measured by diary and questionnaire, in men. *Journal of Studies on Alcohol*. **46**(5): 383–7.

41 Watson HE (1996) Minimal interventions for problem drinkers. *Journal of Substance Misuse*. **1**(2): 107–10.

42 Lockhart SP, Carter YH, Straffen AM *et al.* (1986) Detecting alcohol consumption as a cause of emergency general medical admissions. *Journal of the Royal Society of Medicine.* **79**: 132–6.

43 Watson HE (1993) Minimal interventions for problem drinkers: an evaluation of effectiveness and an analysis of the the nurse's role, Ch 6. University of Strathclyde PhD Thesis.

44 Whitehead TP, Clarke CA and Whitehead AGW (1978) Biological and haematological markers of alcohol intake. *Lancet.* **12**: 978–81.

45 Rollnick S (1997) Whither motivational interviewing? *Journal of Substance Misuse.* **2**(1): 1–2.

46 Watson HE (1993) Minimal interventions for problem drinkers: an evaluation of effectiveness and an analysis of the the nurse's role, Ch 8. University of Strathclyde PhD Thesis.

47 Cooper DB (1994) Problem drinking. *Nursing Times.* **90**(14): 36–9.

Chapter 12: To learn more

Hartz C, Plant M and Watt M (1990) *Alcohol and Health: a handbook for nurses, midwives and health visitors.* The Medical Council on Alcoholism, London.

Hester RK and Miller WR (eds) (1995) *Handbook of Alcoholism Treatment Approaches: effective alternatives* (2nd edn). Allyn and Bacon, Inc., Boston.

Journal of Substance Use (2000) *Special Issue: Alcohol Policies and Developing Countries.* **5**(1) Radcliffe Medical Press, Oxford.

Plant M, Single E and Stockwell T (eds) (1997) *Alcohol: minimising the harm*, Ch 3. Free Association Books, London.

Tracey TJ, Tebutt J and Mattick RP (1995) *Treatment Approaches for Alcohol and Drug Dependence: an introductory guide.* Wiley, Chichester.

Chapter 13

1 Kosten TR and McCance-Katz E (1995) New pharmacotherapies. In *Review of Psychiatry* (eds JM Oldham and MB Riba). American Psychiatric Press, Washington, DC.

2 Carroll K and Rounsaville B (1995) Psychosocial treatments. In *Review of Psychiatry* (eds JM Oldham and MB Riba). American Psychiatric Press, Washington, DC.

3 Prochaska JO, DiClemente CC, Norcross JC (1992) In search of how people change: applications to addictive behaviors. *American Psychologist.* **47**: 1102–14.

4 Brehm SS and Brehm JW (1981) *Psychological Reactance: a theory of freedom and control.* Academic Press, New York.

5 Miller WR and Rollnick S (1991) *Motivational Interviewing: preparing people to change addictive behavior.* Guilford Press, New York.

6 Miller WR, Taylor CA and West JC (1980) Focused versus broad-spectrum behavior therapy for problem drinkers. *Journal of Clinical and Consulting Psychology.* **48**: 590–601.

7 Miller WR and Sovereign RG (1989) The check-up: a model for early intervention in addictive behaviours. In *Addictive Behaviours: prevention and early intervention* (eds T Løberg, WR Miller, PE Nathanm *et al.*), p. 219–31. Swets and Zeitlinger, Amsterdam.

8 Rogers C (1957) The necessary and sufficient conditions for therapeutic personality change. *Journal of Consulting Psychology.* **21**: 95–103.

9 Valle SK (1981) Interpersonal funtioning of alcoholism counsellors and treatment outcome. *Journal of Studies on Alcohol.* **42**: 783–90.

10 Bern DJ (1972) Self-perception theory. In *Advances in Experimental Social Psychology*, Vol. 6 (ed L Berkowitz). Academic Press, New York.

11 Rokeach M (1973) *The Nature of Human Values.* Free Press, New York.

12 Bien T, Miller WR and Burroughs JM (1993) Motivational interviewing with alcohol outpatients. *Behavioral and Cognitive Psychotherapy.* **21**: 347–56.

13 Brown J and Miller WR (1993) Impact of motivational interviewing on participation and outcome in residential alcoholism treatment. *Psychology of Addictive Behaviors.* **7**: 211–18.

14 Project MATCH Research Group (1997) Matching alcoholism treatments to client heterogeneity: Project MATCH post-treatment drinking outcomes. *Journal of Studies on Alcohol.* **58**: 7–29.

15 Noonan WC and Moyers TB (1997) Motivational interviewing: a review. *Journal of Substance Misuse.* **2**: 8–16.

16 Project MATCH Research Group (1998) Therapist effects in three treatments for alcohol problems. *Psychotherapy Research.* **8**: 455–74.

17 Moyers TB and Yahne CE (1998) Motivational interviewing in substance abuse treatment: negotiating roadblocks. *Journal of Substance Misuse.* **3**: 30–3.

Chapter 13: To learn more

The seminal text in the field of motivational interviewing:
Miller WR and Rollnick S (1991) *Motivational Interviewing: preparing people to change addictive behavior.* Guilford Press, New York.

A how-to manual for using motivational interviewing as a stand-alone treatment:
Miller WR, Zweban A, DiClemente CC *et al.* (1992) *Motivational Enhancement Therapy Manual: a clinical research guide for therapists treating individuals with alcohol abuse and dependence.* NIAAA, Rockville, MD. Available from: NIAAA Distribution Center, PO Box 10686, Rockville, MD 20849-0686, USA.

A series of videotapes demonstrating William Miller, Stephen Rollnick and others using motivational interviewing in a variety of settings:
Videotapes. *Motivational Interviewing Professional Training Videotape Series 1998.* European format available from the European Addiction Training Institute, Stadhouderskade 125, 1074 AV Amsterdam, The Netherlands. Telephone: 31-20-675-2041. Available in US version through Delilah Yao, Department of Psychology, University of New Mexico, Albuquerque, NM 87131, USA.

Chapter 14

1 Howard BAM, Harrison S, Carver V *et al.* (eds) (1993) *Alcohol and Drug Problems: a practical guide for counsellors.* Addiction Research Foundation, Toronto.
2 Grant M and Hodgson R (eds) (1991) *Responding to Drug and Alcohol Problems in the Community.* World Health Organization, Geneva.
3 Mattick RP and Jarvis T (1994) A summary of recommendations for the management of alcohol problems: the Quality Assurance in the Treatment of Drug Dependence Project. *Drug and Alcohol Review.* **13**: 145–55.
4 Hyams G, Cartwright A and Spratley T (1996) Engagement in alcohol treatment: the client's experience of, and satisfaction with, the assessment interview. *Addiction Research.* **4**(2): 105–23.
5 Clancy C and Coyne P (1997) Specialist assessment in a multidisciplinary setting. In *Addiction Nursing Perspectives on Professional and Clinical Practice* (eds H Rasnool and M Gafoor). Stanley Thornes, Cheltenham.
6 Rollnick S, Heather N and Bell A (1992) Negotiating behaviour change in medical settings: the development of brief motivational interviewing. *Journal of Mental Health.* **1**: 25–37.
7 Lettieri DJ, Nelson JE and Sayers MA (eds) (1985) *Treatment Assessment Research Instruments.* DHSS publication No. ADM 85, 1380. National Institute on Alcohol Abuse and Alcoholism, Rockville, MD.
8 Project MATCH Research Group (1997) Matching alcoholism treatments to client heterogeneity: Project MATCH post-treatment drinking outcomes. *Journal of Studies on Alcohol.* **58**: 7–29.
9 Stockwell T, Murphy D and Hodgson R (1983) The Severity of Alcohol Dependence Questionnaire: its use, reliability and validity. *British Journal of Addiction.* **78**(2): 145–55.
10 Cooper DB (1994) *Alcohol Home Detoxification and Assessment.* Radcliffe Medical Press, Oxford.
11 Raistrick D, Bradshaw J, Tober G *et al.* (1994) Development of the Leeds Dependence Questionnaire (LDQ): a questionnaire to measure alcohol and opiate dependence in the context of a treatment evaluation package. *Addiction.* **89**: 563–72.

Chapter 14: To learn more

For more information on assessment from a medical perspective:
Royal College of General Practitioners (1986) *Alcohol: a balanced view.* RCGP, London.
Anderson P (1990) *Management of Drinking Problems.* World Health Organization, Geneva.

For a nursing perspective on assessment:
Kennedy J and Faugier J (1989) *Drug and Alcohol Dependency Nursing.* Heinemann, Oxford.

For a counselling perspective:
Howard BAM, Harrison S, Carver V *et al.* (eds) (1993) *Alcohol and Drug Problems: a practical guide for counsellors.* Addiction Research Foundation, Toronto.

Chapter 15

1 World Health Organization (1994) *Lexicon of Alcohol and Drug Terms.* WHO, Geneva.

2 World Health Organization (1993) *WHO Expert Committee on Drug Dependence.* Technical Report Series 28. WHO, Geneva.

3 Foy A (1991) Drug withdrawal: a selective review. *Drug and Alcohol Review.* **10**: 204–14.

4 Williams HI and Rundell OH (1981) Altered sleep physiology in chronic alcoholics: reversal with abstinence. *Alcoholism Clinical and Experimental Research.* **5**: 318–25.

5 Commonwealth Department of Human Services and Health (1994) *Handbook for Medical Practitioners and other Health Workers on Alcohol and other Drug Problems.* Australian Government Publishing Service, Canberra.

6 Stockwell T, Murphy D and Hodgson R (1983) The Severity of Alcohol Dependence Questionnaire: its use, reliability and validity. *British Journal of Addiction.* **78**: 145–56.

7 Cooper DB (1994) *Alcohol Home Detoxification and Assessment.* Radcliffe Medical Press, Oxford.

8 Sullivan J, Sykora K, Schneiderman J *et al.* (1989) Assessment of alcohol withdrawal: the revised Clinical Institute Withdrawal Assessment Scale (CIWA-AR). *British Journal of Addiction.* **84**: 1353–7.

9 Green L and Gossop M (1988) Effects of information on the opiate withdrawal syndrome. *British Journal of Addiction.* **83**: 305–9.

10 Alterman AI, Hayashida M and O'Brian CP (1988) Treatment response and safety of ambulatory medical detoxification. *Journal of Studies on Alcohol.* **49**(2): 160–6.

11 Hayashida M, Alterman AL, McLellan AT *et al.* (1989) Comparative effectiveness and costs of inpatient and outpatient detoxification of patients with mild-to-moderate alcohol withdrawal syndrome. *New England Journal of Medicine.* **320**(6): 358–65.

12 Haigh R and Hibbert G (1990) Where and when to detoxify single homeless drinkers. *British Medical Journal.* **301**(6756): 848–9.

13 Whitfield CL, Thompson G, Lamb A *et al.* (1978) Detoxification of 1024 alcoholic patients without psychoactive drugs. *Journal of the American Medical Association.* **239**(14): 1409–10.

14 Pederson C (1986) Hospital admissions from a non-medical detoxification unit. *Alcohol and Drug Review.* **5**: 133–7.

15 Bartu AE and Saunders W (1994) Domiciliary versus inpatient detoxification for problem drinkers. *Australian Journal of Advanced Nursing.* **11**(4): 12–18.

16 Stockwell T, Bolt E and Hooper J (1986) Detoxification from alcohol at home managed by general practitioners. *British Medical Journal.* **292**: 733–5.

17 Bartu AE (1991) Guidelines for the management of alcohol-related withdrawal symptoms in the home. *Australian Nurses Journal.* **21**(4): 12–13.

Chapter 15: To learn more

Commonwealth Department of Human Services and Health (1994) *Handbook for Medical Practitioners and other Health Workers on Alcohol and other Drug Problems.* Australian Government Publishing Service, Canberra.

Cooper DB (1994) *Alcohol Home Detoxification and Assessment.* Radcliffe Medical Press, Oxford.

Frank L and Pead J (1995) *New Concepts in Drug Withdrawal.* Monograph No. 4. Department of Public Health and Community Medicine, University of Melbourne, Victoria.

Novak H, Ritchie B, Murphy M *et al.* (1997) *Nursing Care of Drug and Alcohol Problems.* Drug and Alcohol Department, Central Area Sydney Health Service.

Chapter 16

1 Mattick RP, Baillie A, Grenyer B *et al.* (1993) *An Outline for the Management of Alcohol Problems: quality assurance project.* National Drug Strategy, Monograph Series No. 20. Australian Government Publishing Service, Canberra.

2 Heather N and Tebbutt J (1989) *The Effectiveness of Treatment for Drug and Alcohol Problems.* National Campaign Against Drug Abuse, Monograph Series No. 11. Commonwealth Department of Community Services and Health, Australian Government Publishing Service, Canberra.

3 Institute of Medicine (1990) *Broadening the Base of Treatment for Alcohol Problems.* National Academy Press, Washington, DC.

4 Brewer C (1993) Recent developments in disulphiram treatment. *Alcohol and Alcoholism.* **28**: 382–95.

5 Hughes JC and Cook CH (1997) The efficacy of disulphiram: a review of outcome studies. *Addiction.* **92**(4): 381–95.

6 Wilde M and Wagstaff A (1997) Acamprosate: a review of its pharmacology and clinical potential in the management of alcohol dependence after detoxification. *Drugs.* **53**(6): 1039–53.

7 AA World Series, Inc. (1988) *Alcoholics Anonymous: the big book* (3rd edn). AA, New York.

8 Egan G (1990) *The Skilled Helper: a systematic approach to effective helping.* Brooks/Cole, California.

9 Miller WR and Rollnick S (1991) *Motivational Interviewing: preparing people to change addictive behavior.* Guilford Press, New York.

10 Lindstrom L (1992) *Managing Alcoholism: matching clients to treatment.* Oxford University Press, New York.

11 Project MATCH Research Group (1997) Matching alcoholism treatments to client heterogeneity: Project MATCH post-treatment drinking outcomes. *Journal of Studies on Alcohol.* **58**: 7–29.

12 Noonan WC and Moyers TB (1997) Motivational interviewing. *Journal of Substance Misuse.* **2**(1): 8–16.

Chapter 16: To learn more

Jarvis T, Tebbutt J and Mattick R (1995) *Treatment Approaches for Alcohol and Drug Dependence*. John Wiley and Sons Ltd, Chichester.

Mattick RP, Baillie A, Grenyer B *et al.* (1993) *An Outline for the Management of Alcohol Problems: quality assurance project*. National Drug Strategy, Monograph Series No. 20. Australian Government Publishing Service, Canberra.

Chapter 17

1 Health Resources and Services Administration (HRSA) (1996) Interdisciplinary training for integrated health care systems in the health workforce. *Newslink: a review of HRSA's Bureau of Health Professions Research and Analysis Activities*. **2**(2): 1.

2 Shugers DA, O'Neil EH, Bader JD (eds) (1991) *Health America: practitioners for 2005, an agenda for action for US health professional schools*. The Pew Health Professions Commission, Durham.

3 McEwen M (1994) Promoting interdisciplinary collaboration. *Nursing and Health Care*. **15**(6): 304–5.

4 Naegle M (1994) *SAEN (Substance Abuse Education in Nursing)*. Volume 1, Module 111.5, p. 186. National League for Nursing Press, New York.

5 Klein JT (1990) *Interdisciplinarity: history, theory and practice*. Wayne State University Press, Detroit.

6 Burke K (1990) Conclusion: the integrative core. In *Interdisciplinarity: history, theory and practice* (ed JT Klein), p. 182. Wayne State University Press, Detroit.

7 Sands RG, Stafford J, McClelland M (1990) 'I beg to differ': conflict in the interdisciplinary team. *Social Work in Health Care*. **14**(3): 55–72.

8 Katzenbach JR and Smith DK (1993) *The Wisdom of Teams* (1st edn). Harper Collins, New York.

9 Marcus LJ, Dorn BC, Kritek PB *et al.* (1995) *Renegotiating Health Care*. Jossey-Bass, San Francisco.

Chapter 17: To learn more

Hackman RJ (ed) (1990) *Groups That Work (And Those That Don't)*. Jossey-Bass, San Francisco.

Katzenbach JR and Smith DK (1993) *The Wisdom of Teams* (1st edn). Harper Collins, New York.

Klein JT (1990) *Interdisciplinarity: history, theory and practice*. Wayne State University Press, Detroit.

Larson CE and LaFasto FM (1989) *Teamwork: what must go right/what can go wrong*. Sage Publications, Newbury Park, CA.

Peters T (1987) *Thriving on Chaos*. Alfred A Knopf, New York.

Peters TJ and Waterman Jr. RH (1982) *In Search of Excellence*. Harper & Row, New York.

Chapter 18

1 *The New Collins Dictionary and Thesaurus* (1987) Harper Collins, Glasgow.
2 United Kingdom Central Council for Nursing, Midwifery and Health Visiting (UKCC) (1999) *Practitioner–Client Relationships and the Prevention of Abuse. Section 5: The professional context.* UKCC, London.
3 United Kingdom Central Council for Nursing, Midwifery and Health Visiting (UKCC) (1999) *Practitioner–Client Relationships and the Prevention of Abuse. Section 7: The value of the individual.* UKCC, London.
4 Cooper DB (1994) *Alcohol Home Detoxification and Assessment.* Radcliffe Medical Press, Oxford.

Chapter 19

1 Robinson J (1988) *Jancis Robinson on the Demon Drink*, p. 118. Mitchell Beazley, London.
2 Reported by Oliver MW (1873) *Source*: http://home.mho.net/coco/drinking.htm, http://www.trail.com/~coco/alcohol–use–and–abuse.htm
3 Reported by Mullerus M (1699) *Source*: http://home.mho.net/coco/drinking.htm, http://www.trail.com/~coco/alcohol–use–and–abuse.htm
4 Reported by Gunn JC (1859) *Source*: http://home.mho.net/coco/drinking.htm, http://www.trail.com/~coco/alcohol–use–and–abuse.htm
5 Reported by Hartshorne H (1871) *Source*: http://home.mho.net/coco/drinking.htm, http://www.trail.com/~coco/alcohol–use–and–abuse.htm
6 Reported by Chase AW (1881) *Source*: http://home.mho.net/coco/drinking.htm, http://www.trail.com/~coco/alcohol–use–and–abuse.htm
7 Reported by Chase AW (1902) *Source*: http://home.mho.net/coco/drinking.htm, http://www.trail.com/~coco/alcohol–use–and–abuse.htm
8 Reported by Richardson JG (1909) *Source*: http://home.mho.net/coco/drinking.htm, http://www.trail.com/~coco/alcohol–use–and–abuse.htm
9 Cooper DB (1994) *Alcohol Home Detoxification and Assessment.* Radcliffe Medical Press, Oxford.
10 Kranzier HR, Modesto-Iowe V, Nuwayser ES *et al.* (1998) Sustained-release naltrexone for alcoholism treatment: a preliminary study. *Alcohol Clinical and Experimental Research.* **22**(5): 1074–9.
11 Sowerby MG (1998) Vitamin replacement for problem drinkers [editorial]. *Journal of Substance Misuse.* **3**(3): 131–2.
12 Cook CCH, Hallwood PM and Thomson AD (1998) B vitamin deficiency and neuropsychiatric syndrome in alcohol misuse. *Alcohol and Alcoholism.* **33**(4): 317–36.
13 Lieber CS (1995) Medical disorders of alcoholism. *New England Journal of Medicine.* **333**: 1054–65.
14 Nine O'Clock News, BBC, 27 October 1999.
15 Home Office (1999) *Under-age Drinking in Public.* Home Office, London.
16 Department of Health (1999) Statistical bulletin: *Statistics on Alcohol: 1976 onwards.* DoH, London.

17 Cooper DB (2000) *The person with dependency problems.* In *Nursing Practice – Hospital and Home: the adult* (eds MF Alexander, JN Fawcett and PJ Runciman), pp. 980–1. Harcourt Brace, Edinburgh.

18 Jensen TK, Hjollund NHJ, Henriksen TB *et al.* (1998) Does moderate alcohol consumption affect fertility? Follow-up study among couples planning first pregnancy. *British Medical Journal.* **317**(7157): 505–10.

19 Purohit V (1998) Moderate alcohol consumption and estrogen levels in postmenopausal women: a review. *Alcoholism Clinical and Experimental Research.* **22**(5): 994–7.

20 Brazier C, Thomas M and Bradleigh L (1998) Creating a much needed balance. *Alcohol Concern Magazine.* **13**(2): 14–17.

21 Hemmingsson T and Lundberg I (1998) Work control, work demands and work social support in relation to alcoholism in young men. *Alcoholism Clinical and Experimental Research.* **22**(4): 921–7.

22 Alcohol Concern (1999) *Measure for Measure: a framework for alcohol policy.* Alcohol Concern, London.

23 Department of Health (1992) *Health of the Nation.* DoH, London.

24 Department of Health (1999) *Saving Lives: our healthier nation.* The Stationery Office, London.

25 Public Opinion Survey on Drink Driving. *Bella Magazine.* 9 March 1999.

26 British Medical Association (1996) *Driving Impairment Through Alcohol and Other Drugs.* BMA, London.

27 Department of the Environment. Transport and Regions (1998) *Combating drink driving: next steps. A consultative paper.* The Stationery Office, London.

28 Morgan G (1999) Drinking and driving legislation: the need for targeted prevention programmes. *Alcoholism.* **18**(4): 1–3.

29 Frankfurter Rundschau, 5 September 1999. *European Alcohol News Digest.* Eurocare. 28 October 1999. http://www.eurocare.org.eronews.htm

30 Dr Miquel Angel Torres Hernández, Socidrogalcohol. *European Alcohol News Digest.* Eurocare. 28 October 1999. http://www.eurocare.org.eronews.htm

31 House of Commons Hansard Debates for 11 May 1999.

32 Department of Health press release. *Government announces timetable for new strategy to tackle alcohol misuse.* 26 May 1999. DoH, London.

33 Department of Health and Social Security and the Welsh Office (1979) *The Pattern and Range of Services for Problem Drinkers: report of the Advisory Committee on Alcoholism.* DHSS and Welsh Office, London.

34 Department of Health and Social Security and the Welsh Office (1979) *Advisory Committee on Alcoholism: report on education and training.* DHSS and Welsh Office, London.

35 Department of Health and Social Security and the Welsh Office (1978) *Advisory Committee on Alcoholism: report on prevention.* DHSS and Welsh Office, London.

Chapter 19: To learn more

Addictions Forum
c/o Alcohol and Health Research Centre
City Hospital
Greenbank Drive
Edinburgh
EH10 5SB
UK
Tel: (+44) (0) 131 536 6189
Fax: (+44) (0) 131 536 6215

Alcohol Concern
Waterbridge House
32–36 Loman Street
London
SE1 0EE
UK
Tel: (+44) (0) 207 928 7377
Tel Bookshop: (+44) (0) 207 928 7377
E-mail: alccon@popmail.dircon.co.uk
Web page: http://www.alcoholconcern.org.uk

Alcohol Education and Research Council
Abell House
John Islip Street
London
SW1P 4HL
UK
Tel: (+44) (0) 207 217 5276

European Addiction Training Institute (EATI)
Stadhouderskade 125
1074 AV Amsterdam
Netherlands
Tel: (+31) 20 675 2041
Fax: (+31) 20 676 4591
E-mail: info@eati.org
Web page: http://www.eati.org

International Council on Alcohol and Addiction (ICAA)
Case postale 189
1001 Lausanne
Switzerland
Tel: (+41) 21 320 98 65
Fax: (+41) 21 320 98 17
E-mail: icaa@pingnet.ch
Web page: http://www.icaa.ch

Institute of Alcohol Studies
Alliance House
12 Caxton Street
London
SW1H 0QS
UK
Tel: (+44) (0) 207 222 5880
Fax: (+44) (0) 207 222 4001
Web page: http://www.ias.org.uk

Medical Council on Alcoholism (MCA)
3 St Andrews Place
London
NW1 4LB
UK
Tel: (+44) (0) 207 487 4445
Fax: (+44) (0) 207 935 4479
E-mail: MCA@medicouncilalco.demon.co.uk
Web page: http://www.medicouncilalco.demon.co.uk

National Nurses Society on Addiction (NNSA)
4101 Lake Boone Trail
Suite 201
Raleigh
North Carolina 27607-7506
USA
Tel: (+1) 919 783 5817
Fax: (+1) 919 787 4916
Web page: http://www.nnsa.org

Nursing Council on Alcohol and Drugs (NCAD)
Parkholme
Ashreigney
Chulmleigh
Devon
EX18 7LY
UK
Tel: (+44) (0) 1769 520 577
Fax: (+44) (0) 8700 562 375
E-mail: david.b.cooper@ashreigney.demon.co.uk

Web pages

British Medical Association
http://www.bma.org.uk

Dual Diagnosis
http://pobox.com/~dualdiagnosis

ENB Health Care Database
http://www.enb.org.uk/hcd.htm

Healthgate
http://www.healthgate.com

Dr Stanton Peele Web Site
http://frw.uva.nl/cedro/peele

UK Public Libraries
http://dspace.dial.pipex.co/town/square/ac940/ukpublib.html/

UKCC
http://www.healthworks.co.uk/hw/orgs/ukcc.html

Virtual clearinghouse for information on alcohol and drugs
http://www.atod.org

World Health Organization (WHO) Newsletter
http://www.who.ch/newsletter/whonewsletter.html

WHO/Cochrane Site
http://hiru.mcmaster.ca/cochrane/

Index